Breast Cancer Imaging I

Guest Editors

RAKESH KUMAR, MD
SANDIP BASU, MD
ABASS ALAVI, MD,
MD (Hon), PhD (Hon), DSc (Hon)

PET CLINICS

www.pet.theclinics.com

Consulting Editor
ABASS ALAVI, MD,
MD (Hon), PhD (Hon), DSc (Hon)

July 2009 • Volume 4 • Number 3

SAUNDERS an imprint of ELSEVIER, Inc.

W.B. SAUNDERS COMPANY
A Division of Elsevier Inc.

1600 John F. Kennedy Boulevard • Suite 1800 • Philadelphia, Pennsylvania 19103-2899

http://www.theclinics.com

PET CLINICS Volume 4, Number 3
July 2009 ISSN 1556-8598, ISBN 10: 1-4377-0964-8, ISBN-13: 978-1-4377-0964-3

Editor: Barton Dudlick

PET Clinics (ISSN 1556-8598) is published quarterly by Elsevier Inc., 360 Park Avenue South, New York, NY 10010-1710. Months of issue are January, April, July, and October. Periodicals postage paid at New York, NY, and additional mailing offices. Subscription prices per year are $196.00 (US individuals), $279.00 (US institutions), $97.00 (US students), $223.00 (Canadian individuals), $312.00 (Canadian institutions), $118.00 (Canadian students), $237.00 (foreign individuals), $312.00 (foreign institutions), and $118.00 (foreign students). To receive student and resident rate, orders must be accompanied by name of affiliated institution, date of term, and the signature of program/residency coordinator on institution letterhead. Orders will be billed at individual rate until proof of status is received. Foreign air speed delivery is included in all Clinics subscription prices. All prices are subject to change without notice. POSTMASTER: Send address changes to PET Clinics, Elsevier Health Sciences Division, Subscription Customer Service, 3251 Riverport Lane, Maryland Heights, MO 63043. **Customer Service: 1-800-654-2452 (U.S. and Canada); 314-447-8871 (outside U.S. and Canada). Fax: 314-447-8029. E-mail: journalscustomerservice-usa@elsevier.com (for print support); journalsonlinesupport-usa@elsevier.com (for online support).**

Reprints. For copies of 100 or more of articles in this publication, please contact the Commercial Reprints Department, Elsevier Inc., 360 Park Avenue South, New York, NY 10010-1710. Tel.: 212-633-3812; Fax: 212-462-1935; E-mail: reprints@elsevier.com.

Printed and bound in the United Kingdom
Transferred to Digital Print 2011

Contributors

CONSULTING EDITOR

ABASS ALAVI, MD, MD (Hon), PhD (Hon), DSc (Hon)
Professor of Radiology, Department
of Radiology, Division of Nuclear Medicine,
Hospital of University of Pennsylvania,
University of Pennsylvania School of Medicine,
Philadelphia, Pennsylvania

GUEST EDITORS

RAKESH KUMAR, MD
Associate Professor, Department of Nuclear
Medicine, All India Institute of Medical Sciences,
New Delhi, India

SANDIP BASU, MD
Scientist, Radiation Medicine Centre, BARC,
Mumbai, India

ABASS ALAVI, MD, MD (Hon), PhD (Hon), DSc (Hon)
Professor of Radiology, Department of Radiology,
Division of Nuclear Medicine, Hospital of
University of Pennsylvania, University of
Pennsylvania School of Medicine, Philadelphia,
Pennsylvania

AUTHORS

ABEER AL-MULLAH, MD
Chief, Department of Medical Imaging,
King Fahd Specialist Hospital, Dammam,
Saudi Arabia

ABASS ALAVI, MD, MD (Hon), PhD (Hon), DSc (Hon)
Professor of Radiology, Department of Radiology,
Division of Nuclear Medicine, Hospital of
University of Pennsylvania, University of
Pennsylvania School of Medicine, Philadelphia,
Pennsylvania

NOOR M. ALNAIMY, MD
Women's Imaging Consultant and Academic
Coordinator, Medical Imaging Department,
King Fahad Specialist Hospital, Dammam,
Saudi Arabia

SUSAN BAHL, MD
Department of Surgery, University of Pennsylvania
School of Medicine, Philadelphia, Pennsylvania

SANDIP BASU, MD
Scientist, Radiation Medicine Centre, BARC,
Mumbai, India

BRIAN J. CZERNIECKI, MD, PhD
Department of Surgery, University of
Pennsylvania School of Medicine, Philadelphia,
Pennsylvania

CHANDAN J. DAS, MD
Senior Radiologist, Department of Radiology,
All India Institute of Medical Sciences,
New Delhi, India

WILLIAM B. EUBANK, MD
Associate Professor of Radiology, Department
of Radiology, Puget Sound VA Health Care
System, Seattle, Washington

SMRITI HARI, MD
Assistant Professor of Radiology, Department
of Radio-Diagnosis, All India Institute of Medical
Sciences, New Delhi, India

NUHA KHOUMAIS, MD
Clinical Fellow, Department of Medical Imaging, University of British Columbia; BC Cancer Agency, Vancouver, British Columbia, Canada

RAKESH KUMAR, MD
Associate Professor, Department of Nuclear Medicine, All India Institute of Medical Sciences, New Delhi, India

JEAN H. LEE, MD
Assistant Professor Radiology, Department of Radiology, University of Washington and Seattle Cancer Care Alliance, Seattle, Washington

DAVID A. MANKOFF, MD, PhD
Professor of Radiology, Department of Radiology, University of Washington and Seattle Cancer Care Alliance, Seattle, Washington

CHETAN PATEL, MD
Department of Nuclear Medicine, All India Institute of Medical Sciences, New Delhi, India

NEERJA RANI, PhD
Demonstrator, Department of Anatomy, All India Institute of Medical Sciences, New Delhi, India

ROBERT E. ROSES, MD
Department of Surgery, University of Pennsylvania School of Medicine, Philadelphia, Pennsylvania

SANJAY THULKAR, MD
Associate Professor of Radiology, Dr BR Ambedkar Institute Rotary Cancer Hospital, All India Institute of Medical Sciences, New Delhi, India

SUSAN WEINSTEIN, MD
Associate Professor, Division of Breast Imaging, University of Pennsylvania Medical Center, Philadelphia, Pennsylvania

Contents

Present Role of Mammography/Digital Mammography in Breast Cancer Management   **213**

Sanjay Thulkar and Smriti Hari

> Mammography is the primary breast imaging modality. Its major role is in breast can-
> cer screening. Other indications of mammography are referred to as "diagnostic
> mammography," and these include evaluation of patients with symptomatic breast
> diseases, search of the occult primary cancer, preoperative evaluation, and follow-
> up of patients with breast cancer. Other imaging modalities compliment, but do not
> generally replace, mammography. Digital mammography has further improved the
> technical capabilities of mammography.

Role of Ultrasonography in Breast Cancer Imaging   **227**

Noor M. Alnaimy and Nuha Khoumais

> Familiarity with breast ultrasound in terms of technique, indications, anatomy, and
> interpretation is vital for proper breast examinations. Ultrasound is a basic method
> of approaching breast masses and an important tool in interventional breast proce-
> dures. Combination of mammogram and ultrasound examinations when indicated is
> an effective method in increasing rate of cancer detection. Second-look ultrasound
> is an effective method to localize lesions missed in the initial scanning.

Evolving Role of MRI in Breast Cancer Imaging   **241**

Susan Weinstein

> Breast MRI is a useful adjunctive tool to mammography. In the past 2 decades, con-
> trast-enhanced breast MRI has become an integral component of breast imaging. In
> patients with known breast cancer, breast MRI can assess the extent of disease, in-
> cluding multifocal tumors and chest wall invasion. Improvements in MRI technology
> have resulted in improved ability for diagnosing mammographically and clinically oc-
> cult breast cancer. With the use of contrast, the sensitivity of breast MRI for assess-
> ing invasive breast cancer approaches 100%, although specificity is lower. The
> clinical indications for the use of breast MRI will continue to evolve and expand.

FDG-PET Dynamic Contrast-Enhanced CT in the Management of Breast Cancer   **255**

Chandan J. Das, Abeer Al-Mullah, and Rakesh Kumar

> Breast cancer is a complex disease and molecular imaging may contribute to better
> management through providing new insight for early detection. Fluorodeoxyglucose
> (FDG)-PET/CT has made great strides as a functional anatomic technique and re-
> cently gained attention in the diagnosis, staging, and follow-up of breast cancer.
> FDG-PET and CT complement each other's strengths in integrated FDGPET/CT.
> One-stop-shop whole-body FDG-PET/CT coupled with integrated FDG-PET/CT
> mammography has also been advocated.

PET Clinics

THE CLINICS ARE NOW AVAILABLE ONLINE!

Access your subscription at:
www.theclinics.com

GOAL STATEMENT

The goal of the *PET Clinics* is to keep practicing radiologists and radiology residents up to date with current clinical practice in positron emission tomography by providing timely articles reviewing the state of the art in patient care.

ACCREDITATION

PET Clinics is planned and implemented in accordance with the Essential Areas and Policies of the Accreditation Council for Continuing Medical Education (ACCME) through the joint sponsorship of the University of Virginia School of Medicine and Elsevier. The University of Virginia School of Medicine is accredited by the ACCME to provide continuing medical education for physicians.

The University of Virginia School of Medicine designates this educational activity for a maximum of 15 *AMA PRA Category 1 Credits*™ for each issue, 60 credits per year. Physicians should only claim credit commensurate with the extent of their participation in the activity.

The American Medical Association has determined that physicians not licensed in the US who participate in this CME activity are eligible for a maximum of 15 *AMA PRA Category 1 Credits*™ for each issue, 60 credits per year.

Category 1 credit can be earned by reading the text material, taking the CME examination online at http://www.theclinics.com/home/cme, and completing the evaluation. After taking the test, you will be required to review any and all incorrect answers. Following completion of the test and evaluation, your credit will be awarded and you may print your certificate.

FACULTY DISCLOSURE/CONFLICT OF INTEREST

The University of Virginia School of Medicine, as an ACCME accredited provider, endorses and strives to comply with the Accreditation Council for Continuing Medical Education (ACCME) Standards of Commercial Support, Commonwealth of Virginia statutes, University of Virginia policies and procedures, and associated federal and private regulations and guidelines on the need for disclosure and monitoring of proprietary and financial interests that may affect the scientific integrity and balance of content delivered in continuing medical education activities under our auspices.

The University of Virginia School of Medicine requires that all CME activities accredited through this institution be developed independently and be scientifically rigorous, balanced and objective in the presentation/discussion of its content, theories and practices.

All authors/editors participating in an accredited CME activity are expected to disclose to the readers relevant financial relationships with commercial entities occurring within the past 12 months (such as grants or research support, employee, consultant, stock holder, member of speakers bureau, etc.). The University of Virginia School of Medicine will employ appropriate mechanisms to resolve potential conflicts of interest to maintain the standards of fair and balanced education to the reader. Questions about specific strategies can be directed to the Office of Continuing Medical Education, University of Virginia School of Medicine, Charlottesville, Virginia.

The faculty and staff of the University of Virginia Office of Continuing Medical Education have no financial affiliations to disclose.

The authors/editors listed below have identified no professional or financial affiliations for themselves or their spouse/partner:
Abass Alavi, MD, MD(Hon), PhD(Hon), DSc(Hon) (Guest Editor); Noor M. Alnaimy, MD; Susan Bahl, MD; Sandip Basu, MD (Guest Editor); Brian J. Czerniecki, MD, PhD; Chandan J. Das, MD; Barton Dudlick (Acquisitions Editor); William B. Eubank, MD; Smriti Hari, MD; Nuha Khoumais, MD; Rakesh Kumar, MD (Guest Editor); Jean H. Lee, MD; Chetan Patel, MD; Neerja Rani, PhD; Patrice Rehm, MD (Test Author); Robert E. Roses, MD; Sanjay Thulkar, MD; and Susan P. Weinstein, MD.

The authors/editors listed below identified the following professional or financial affiliations for themselves or their spouse/partner:
Abeer Al-Mullah, MD is employed and is a consultant at the King Fahad Specialist Hospital-Dammam KSA.
David A. Mankoff, MD, PhD is an industry funded research/investigator for Pfizer and Merck.

Disclosure of Discussion of Non-FDA Approved Uses for Pharmaceutical Products and/or Medical Devices.
The University of Virginia School of Medicine, as an ACCME provider, requires that all faculty presenters identify and disclose any off-label uses for pharmaceutical and medical device products. The University of Virginia School of Medicine recommends that each physician fully review all the available data on new products or procedures prior to clinical use.

TO ENROLL

To enroll in the PET Clinics Continuing Medical Education program, call customer service at 1-800-654-2452 or visit us online at www.theclinics.com/home/cme. The CME program is available to subscribers for an additional fee of $175.00.

Preface

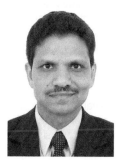

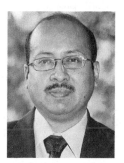

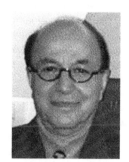

Rakesh Kumar, MD

Sandip Basu, MD

Abass Alavi, MD,
MD (Hon), PhD (Hon), DSc (Hon)

Guest Editors

Breast cancer is the most frequently diagnosed cancer and the second most common cause of death due to cancer in women throughout the world. In 2009, it is estimated that 192,370 new cases of breast cancer will be diagnosed among women and 40,170 patients will die from breast cancer in the United States.[1] While its incidence has increased in the past decades, the overall mortality from this disease has decreased in recent years,[2] mainly because of early diagnosis and better management. In the last decade, the treatment of breast cancer has become less radical as it has become increasingly coupled with primary chemotherapy. Noninvasive imaging plays an important role in early detection of breast cancer and in directing its therapy. Many imaging modalities can be used for the management of breast cancer for making the initial diagnosis, staging, monitoring the treatment response, detecting recurrence, and predicting tumor behavior. This issue of *PET Clinics* on breast cancer is the first part of a two-part series and provides a comprehensive review of multimodality imaging with special emphasis on positron emission tomography (PET) and combination PET and CT (PET/CT) imaging in the context of breast cancer management strategies. Part I provides an overview of mammography, MR imaging, ultrasonography, dynamic multiphase CT, PET–PET/CT, and sentinel lymph node (SLN) biopsy for detection and for staging and restaging in patients with breast cancer. Part II will cover radionuclide imaging of breast cancer response to therapy, other clinical indications for radionuclide breast cancer imaging, and future directions, including molecular imaging and radiotherapy treatment planning.

Mammography remains the primary imaging modality for breast cancer screening.[3] Early detection of the cancer has been shown to reduce breast cancer deaths in randomized controlled trials of mammography in women aged 50 to 69 years. Current breast cancer screening includes mammography and clinical examination. Mammography offers the best ratio of benefits to side effects of any screening method tested to date. Although mammography is an effective imaging tool, it has its limitations, which include moderate sensitivity and specificity. This has led to the development of alternative imaging tools for distinguishing benign from malignant lesions in the breast. Such tools as digital mammography, ultrasound, MR imaging, optical imaging, and PET have been suggested and the preliminary data demonstrate promise in improving the diagnostic accuracy over film screen mammography alone. Ultrasound and MR imaging are important adjuncts to mammography for both diagnosis and characterization of breast lesions. In the past 2 decades, contrast-enhanced breast MR imaging has become an integral component of breast imaging. Over the years, improvements in MR imaging technology and biopsy capability have enabled diagnoses of mammographically and clinically occult breast cancer. In her article, Weinstein beautifully describes the role of MR imaging in the detection and diagnosis of breast cancer, especially in determining the extent of disease within the breast. MR imaging is more sensitive than mammography in screening high-risk women (ie, those with suspected or proven inherited mutations of the breast cancer genes) and was recently incorporated into the American Cancer Society recommendations for screening of these patients.[4] However, MR imaging significantly increases a woman's risk of being recalled for investigation or surgical biopsy

PET Clin 4 (2009) ix–xi
doi:10.1016/j.cpet.2009.10.005

for false-positive findings. Ultrasonography is one method of choice for guiding breast biopsies of suspected lesion of breast. In their article, Alnaimy and Khoumais explain that ultrasonography plays an important role in approaching breast masses and is a major tool in interventional breast procedures. The role of dynamic contrast-enhanced CT (CECT) in diagnosis is still evolving. The article by Das and colleagues reviews the role of CECT imaging, which can readily provide the required morphologic data while CT perfusion can assess the tumor neovascularity. The perfusion data obtained by dynamic CECT appears to be promising and is likely to have some incremental value over structural and metabolic data provided by flurodeoxyglucose cose (FDG) PET/CT.

Most of the initial PET studies done in fewer patients and with larger primary breast tumors demonstrated a variable sensitivity (range 63%–96%) and specificity (range 75%–100%) of PET and PET/CT in evaluating primary breast lesions.[5–10] However, recent studies done in smaller breast tumors demonstrated lower diagnostic accuracy of PET and PET/CT.[7–10] Despite many advantages of PET/CT, there are certain shortcomings as an imaging tool of primary breast cancer. The review by Kumar and colleagues describes various important causes of false-negative and false-positive PET and PET/CT imaging when used for the diagnosis of primary breast cancer. PET has limited sensitivity in detecting lesions less than 10 mm. This limitation is overcome by use of PET/CT, which has resolution of about 4 mm. Slowly growing and well-differentiated histologic subtypes of breast cancer, such as tubular carcinoma, lobular carcinoma, and in situ carcinoma demonstrate lower FDG uptake as compared with invasive ductal cancer.[7,8] In spite of great successes achieved by FDG-PET imaging in the evaluation of malignant disorders, the test is not specific for cancer. Benign processes, such as infection, inflammation, and granulomatous diseases, appear to have increased glycolysis and are therefore readily visualized by FDG-PET imaging. Recently, positron emission mammography (PEM) has been developed to overcome the limitations of whole-body FDG-PET–PET/CT. Compared with PET–PET/CT, PEM has higher spatial resolution, shorter imaging time, and reduced attenuation. A recent multicenter trial also suggested that PEM may aid in the detection and characterization of both invasive and in situ breast carcinoma.[11] Berg and colleagues[12] reported that 10 of 11 in situ carcinomas were detected by PEM, and 8 of 10 were detected by mammography and ultrasonography. However, utility of PEM, compared with existing breast-imaging methods, needs validation in larger prospective trials.

In breast cancer, lymph node involvement has important prognostic and therapeutic implications. Staging is typically divided into locoregional staging (axillary nodes) and distant or systemic staging (distant metastases). There is no effective noninvasive modality for determining the involvement of the axillary lymph nodes; lymph node dissection fully evaluates the draining lymph nodes. Identifying SLNs for initial sampling and dissection is a well-established procedure for detecting axillary lymph node metastasis from primary breast cancer.[13,14] Roses and colleagues in their review in this issue discuss role of sentinel node mapping in axially lymph node staging in breast cancer. This procedure has been validated through multiple randomized trials and enables more accurate prediction of the presence of axillary metastases. Data from several ongoing clinical trials may better define the role of SLN biopsy before and following neoadjuvant chemotherapy. However, For SLN biopsy to be most useful, PET/CT pre-chemotherapy and SLN biopsy posttherapy may also be required. Clinical trials are underway to determine the utility of this approach. FDG-PET can visualize axillary lymph node metastasis by detecting changes in metabolism before anatomic change appears on CT scan. However PET can miss small axillary metastasis and its sensitivity varies from 79% to 100% and specificity ranges from 66% to 100%.[15] Thus, 18F-FDG-PET is not sufficiently accurate to replace SLN biopsy in patients with early-stage breast cancer. Many investigators reported high specificity of PET–PET/CT in detecting axillary lymph node metastasis, especially in patients with locally advanced breast cancer. In such patients, FDG-PET plays an important role possibly in conjunction with MR imaging. In breast cancer, FDG-PET can be helpful in assessing spread to regional nodal sites other than axilla sites, such as internal mammary chain and interpectoral sites. For detection of distant metastasis, bone scan is most commonly used for bone metastasis detection. However, it has low specificity and limited value in lytic bone metastasis and bone marrow metastasis. FDG-PET and PET/CT are helpful in the detection of bone metastases. FDG-PET is superior to bone scanning in the detection of lytic and intramedullary metastases, but inferior in the detection of primarily osteoblastic lesions.

Recurrent disease is typically categorized as (1) locoregional recurrence, (2) internal mammary and other extra-axial regional lymph node recurrence, and (3) distant metastasis. Significant changes have recently taken place in treatment strategies in clinical practice in patients with recurrent breast cancer.[16,17] These changes stem mainly from improvements in restaging accuracy for FDG-PET and PET/CT compared with conventional imaging in patients suspected of having local or distant recurrence. The detection of more widespread disease by FDG-PET is, particularly in patients, thought to have limited locoregional disease based on conventional imaging. FDG-PET can select patients more appropriately for systemic treatment alone, rather than more aggressive, curative treatments, such as surgery and radiation.[17] In their article, Eubank and colleagues demonstrate the role of FDG-PET imaging in patients with breast cancer for restaging and diagnosis of recurrent and metastatic disease following primary therapy. FDG-PET and PET/CT are useful tools for restaging breast cancer patients who have undergone primary therapy, particularly in those with advanced stages, those with equivocal findings at conventional staging studies, or those who are asymptomatic with elevated tumor markers. The potential of FDG-PET to provide more accurate and earlier detection of breast cancer recurrences will, it is hoped, translate into more effective treatment strategies and better health outcomes for these patients in the future.

Rakesh Kumar, MD
Department of Nuclear Medicine
All India Institute of Medical Sciences
New Delhi, 110029, India

Sandip Basu, MD
Radiation Medicine Centre
BARC, Mumbai, India

Abass Alavi, MD,
MD (Hon), PhD (Hon), DSc (Hon)
Nuclear Medicine Section
Department of Radiology
Hospital of the University of Pennsylvania
3400 Spruce Street
Philadelphia, PA 19104, USA

E-mail addresses:
rkphulia@hotmail.com (R. Kumar)
drsanb@yahoo.com (S. Basu)
abass.alavi@uphs.upenn.edu (A. Alavi)

REFERENCES

1. Jemal A, Siegel R, Ward E, et al. Cancer statistics, 2009. CA Cancer J Clin 2009;59:225–49.
2. Jemal A, Clegg LX, Elizabeth Ward E, et al. Annual report to the nation on the status of cancer, 1975–2001, with a special feature regarding survival. Cancer 2004;101(1):3–27.
3. Elmore JG, Armstrong K, Lehman CD, et al. Screening for breast cancer. JAMA 2005;293:1245–56.
4. Saslow D, Boetes C, Burke W, et al. American Cancer Society guidelines for breast screening with MRI as an adjunct to mammography. CA Cancer J Clin 2007;57:75–89.
5. Wahl RL, Cody RL, Hutchins GD, et al. Primary and metastatic breast carcinoma: initial clinical evaluation with PET with the radiolabeled glucose analogue 2-[F-18]-fluoro-2-deoxy-D-glucose. Radiology 1991; 179:765–70.
6. Adler LP, Crowe JP, al-Kaisi NK, et al. Evaluation of breast masses and axillary lymph nodes with [F-18] 2-deoxy-2-fluoro-D-glucose PET. Radiology 1993;187:743–50.
7. Kumar R, Chauhan A, Zhuang H, et al. Clinicopathologic factors associated with false negative FDG-PET in primary breast cancer. Breast Cancer Res Treat 2006;98(3):267–74.
8. Avril N, Rose CA, Schelling M, et al. Breast imaging with positron emission tomography and fluorine-18 fluorodeoxyglucose: use and limitations. J Clin Oncol 2000;18:3495–502.
9. Kumar R, Loving V, Chauhan A, et al. Dual time point imaging and its potential to improve breast cancer diagnosis with F18-fluorodeoxyglucose positron emission tomography. J Nucl Med 2005;46(11):1819–24.
10. Heusner TA, Kuemmel S, Umutlu L, et al. Breast cancer staging in a single session: whole-body PET/CT mammography. J Nucl Med 2008;49(8):1215–22.
11. Rosen EL, Eubank WB, Mankoff DA. FDG PET, PET/CT, and breast cancer imaging. Radiographics 2007;27(Suppl 1):S215–29.
12. Berg WA, Weinberg IN, Narayanan D, et al. High-resolution fluorodeoxyglucose positron emission tomography with compression ("positron emission mammography") is highly accurate in depicting primary breast cancer. Breast J 2006;12:309–23.
13. Albertini JJ, Lyman GH, Cox C, et al. Lymphatic mapping and sentinel node biopsy in the patient with breast cancer. JAMA 1996;276:1818–22.
14. Kumar R, Jana S, Heiba SI, et al. Retrospective analysis of sentinel node localization in multicentric palpable and non-palpable breast cancer. J Nucl Med 2003;44:7–10.
15. Kumar R, Chauhan A, Zhuang H, et al. FDG-PET positive lymph nodes are highly predictive of metastasis in breast cancer. Nucl Med Commun 2006;27:231–6.
16. Yap CS, Seltzer MA, Schiepers C, et al. Impact of whole-body [F-18]-FDG PET on staging and managing patients with breast cancer: the referring physician's perspective. J Nucl Med 2001;42(9):1334–7.
17. Eubank W, Mankoff D, Bhattacharya M, et al. Impact of [F-18]-Fluorodeoxyglucose PET on defining the extent of disease and management of patients with recurrent or metastatic breast cancer. AJR Am J Roentgenol 2004;183:479–86.

Present Role of Mammography/ Digital Mammography in Breast Cancer Management

Sanjay Thulkar, MD[a],*, Smriti Hari, MD[b]

KEYWORDS
- Mammography • Breast cancer • Management
- Preoperative • Follow up

Mammography is the primary breast imaging modality. Its aim is to detect breast abnormalities, especially those suspicious for breast cancer, before these become clinically apparent. The most important indication of mammography is screening for breast cancer. Mammography is the only modality established as a definitive breast cancer screening tool. This status was achieved after multiple large population-based randomized screening trials, simultaneous evolution of the equipment and technique, developments in the knowledge of the biology and management of breast cancer, and analysis of the long-term results.[1] Sensitivity of screening mammography in detection of breast cancers ranges from 83% to 95%.[2,3] It decreases to variable extent in patients with dense and glandular breast. Detailed discussion of mammographic screening is beyond the scope of this article.

Other indications of mammography, frequently grouped under the heading of "diagnostic mammography," include evaluation of patients with breast symptoms, search of the occult primary tumor in those presenting with metastases, preoperative evaluation of breasts in patients diagnosed with breast cancer, and follow-up patients after surgery. Mammography is not performed in pregnant or lactating women and is generally avoided in women below 30 years of age.[4]

BASIC PHYSICS AND TECHNIQUES

Mammography is a high-contrast and high-resolution radiographic examination of the breasts. The breast tissues are all soft tissues with little inherent contrast among them. This contrast must be highlighted so as to differentiate among various normal and abnormal structures. The spatial resolution of mammography is much higher than that of any other imaging modality. This allows detection and evaluation of the morphology to characterize various breast abnormalities when these are very small. For higher contrast, low kilovolt (peak) radiographs are used. The molybdenum or rhodium anodes used in mammographic x-ray tubes are valuable to produce low-energy x-ray photons, because the characteristic radiations of these metals fulfill the requirements of mammography. Very low energy photons, which are likely to be absorbed in the breast and not contribute to the image formation, are removed using filters at the source of the x-ray beam. The films used for mammography also have narrow x-ray

[a] Department of Radiology, Dr BR Ambedkar Institute Rotary Cancer Hospital, All India Institute of Medical Sciences, New Delhi 110029, India
[b] Department of Radio-diagnosis, All India Institute of Medical Sciences, New Delhi 110029, India
* Corresponding author.
E-mail address: thulkar@hotmail.com (S. Thulkar).

PET Clin 4 (2009) 213–225
doi:10.1016/j.cpet.2009.09.006

exposure latitude and thereby further improve the contrast in the images. Small focal spot of the x-ray tube and high-resolution film-screen combinations improve the spatial resolution of the mammography, which may be up to 15 to 20 lp/mm.

Good breast compression with radiolucent compression paddle is mandatory for mammography. This may make the examination unpleasant to some women; however, it is essential to hold the breast away from the chest wall and stabilize and compress it into the mammographic field. Breast compression results in uniform thickness and hence uniform exposures and densities in most parts of the breast. The overlapping tissues are separated and spread evenly, which improves their visualization. Firm compression of the breast closer to film or image receptor reduces the geometric blur and magnification. Compression also stabilizes the breast and reduces movement blur. Mammography cannot be performed if breast compression is not possible. Such situations may include uncooperative women, presence of a wound, recent surgery, or tender breasts.

In a standard mammographic examination, a pair of mediolateral-oblique and craniocaudal views are obtained for each breasts. These provide two orthogonal images for basic imaging evaluation of the breast. Entire breast cannot be included in any single mammographic view; however, an attempt is always made to include as much of the breast as possible in the images. The skills of the technologists are crucial to correctly position the patient to maximize the

breast tissue included in the image and to provide adequate compression to the breast without making it painful to the patient. Additional mammographic views may sometimes be recommended for further clarifications. Some of these are rolled view, spot compression view (**Fig. 1**), magnification view, axillary tail view, cleavage view, extended craniocaudal view, and straight mediolateral view.

For accurate detection and characterization of breast abnormalities on mammography, good quality control is essential. It is required at several steps: acceptance and periodic maintenance of the equipment, positioning and exposure, film processing, viewing conditions, and the interpretation. The quality control requirements of mammography are probably more stringent than any other imaging modality. Modern mammographic examinations are safe and the mean glandular radiation dose to the breast rarely exceeds 3 mGy per image. With present mammographic equipment, there is little or no radiation-related risk to women over 40 years of age.[5]

DIGITAL MAMMOGRAPHY

Because of the stringent technical requirements of mammography, it was the last imaging technique to go digital. During the initial years of digital mammography, major technical challenges were the building of high-resolution digital detectors, high-resolution and brightness monitors, powerful workstations to handle the data of several and heavy digital images, and high memory

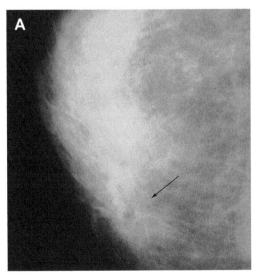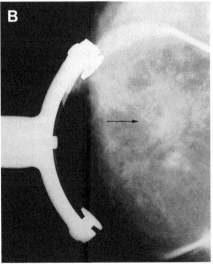

Fig. 1. (*A*) Craniocaudal view of mammogram shows an area of architectural distortion (*arrow*) with no definite mass. (*B*) Rolled spot compression mammographic view of the same area shows underlying spiculated mass (*arrow*) highly suspicious for cancer (BI-RADS category 5).

requirements for storage. With technical developments, these limitations have been overcome to some extent and full-field digital mammography is now gradually replacing the screen-film (conventional) mammography. The technology is still evolving, however, and overall most centers still use screen-film mammography.

The most important component of digital mammography is the digital detector. It converts the x-rays into electronic images and replaces the film. The detector technology is largely vendor specific; however, these can be broadly divided into two types. The indirect digital detectors convert x-rays into light and then into electronic image. These detectors use amorphous silicon, charge-couple devices, or photostimulable phosphors. The direct digital detectors, often called "flat panel detectors," directly convert x-rays into a digital image. These use scintillators of amorphous selenium.[6] The overall design of the mammography unit (including x-ray tube, gantry, compression paddles), technique of performing the mammography, amount of radiation involved, and interpretation and reporting remain similar to those of screen-film mammography.

ADVANTAGES AND APPLICATIONS OF DIGITAL MAMMOGRAPHY

Digital mammography images are available for viewing immediately and the darkroom, which is frequently a major source of image degradation and artifacts, is eliminated. The contrast characteristics and the dynamic range (ability to handle and display the range of gray scale) are better than screen-film mammography. Other advantages of digital mammography are same as those offered by any digital modality. These include postprocessing, such as manipulations of the contrast, brightness, edge enhancement, zoom-pan, and so forth. The digital images are also suitable for better archival, storage, and communication (ie, PACS and telemammography). When compared with screen-film mammography, major limitations of digital mammography are the cost and lower spatial resolution. Full-field digital mammography units are several times more expensive than conventional mammography units. The spatial resolution of current digital mammography systems is about 6 to 8 lp/mm (ie, about half of what is possible with screen-film mammography). Better dynamic range and postprocessing abilities compensate this, however, and does not significantly affect lesion detection and characterization on digital mammography.

Earlier comparative studies reported better cancer detection rates with screen-film mammography than digital mammography.[7,8] Subsequently, both modalities demonstrated similar cancer detection rates.[9] Digital mammography probably offers some advantages in women under 50 years of age and in those with dense breasts.[9,10]

Newer applications of digital mammography are exciting. These include computer-aided detection and diagnosis, digital breast tomosynthesis, and dual-energy contrast-enhanced mammography. Computer-aided detection and diagnosis software highlights the areas of calcifications and masses, which are then carefully assessed by the radiologist. Computer-aided detection and diagnosis decreases the chances of overlooking these abnormalities. It may help inexperienced radiologists, and also act as a second opinion to experienced radiologists.[11] Use of computer-aided detection and diagnosis at screening setup improves cancer detection rates.[12] Digital breast tomosynthesis is a technique in which a moving x-ray tube is used to obtain multiple projections at different depths. The images are reconstructed in the form of sections similar to the CT. This help to distinguish glandular breast tissues from true lesions, especially in dense breasts. The dense glandular tissue in conventional mammography is frequently a source of both false-positives and false-negatives. The overlapping glandular tissue may hide the mass, and in others it may simulate the mass when none exists. Tomosynthesis provides sectional images and improves the accuracy of mammography. It is more useful in characterization of masses and asymmetries than in the evaluation of calcifications.[13] Dual-energy subtraction contrast-enhanced mammography involves intravenous contrast and it can demonstrate some of the cancers when standard mammography findings are suspicious.[14] Both these techniques are investigational at present and clinical studies are expected in future.

MAMMOGRAPHY REPORTING

To achieve uniformity and objectivity in the interpretation and reporting of mammograms, the American College of Radiology has developed standard guidelines that are increasingly being used, called Beast Imaging Reporting and Data System (BI-RADS).[15] The mammographic results or assessments are categorized from BI-RADS 0 to BI-RADS 6, which are primarily aimed for communication of significance of the mammographic findings to the referring physician and to recommend the most appropriate management. BI-RADS category 0 represents incomplete evaluation when repeat mammography, additional views, or investigations, such as ultrasound or MR imaging (but not biopsy), are recommended. Category 1 is normal mammogram and category 2 is definitely benign findings, such as benign calcification or a fat-containing mass. No specific management is required. Category 3 is a probably benign finding with extremely low chances of malignancy. Short-term follow-up is recommended. Category 4 represents findings with low to high concern for malignancy, and category 5 is characteristic mammographic findings with very high probability of malignancy. Biopsy is recommended for both category 4 and 5 lesions. BI-RADS 6 category is used to denote biopsy-proved malignancy when breast imaging is being performed as a part of pretreatment work-up. BI-RADS also incorporate the breast imaging lexicon (ie, standard terms and nomenclature for description, analysis, and interpretation of breast lesions). Originally developed for mammography only, it is now also available for ultrasound and MR imaging examinations of the breast.[16] BI-RADS is still evolving and many consider it as an optimal structured reporting format, which may serve as a model for other imaging modalities. Apart from standardization, such reporting formats also help to minimize the ambiguity from the reports and make the results reproducible and comparable.

MAMMOGRAPHIC FEATURES OF BREAST CANCER

Breast cancer can manifest on mammography in several ways: mass, calcifications, architectural distortion, asymmetry, or any combination of these. Ancillary signs of malignancy, such as lymphadenopathy, breast edema, skin or areolar thickening, or retraction, may be seen in advanced cases. Mammographic abnormalities are not specific for cancer and based on the morphology, these may elicit various degrees of suspicion for breast cancer. Biopsy is mandatory for definitive diagnosis of breast cancer.

Mass is a space-occupying lesion in the breast, which is seen in two views. Lesion seen in only one view is considered a density unless its three-dimensional existence is established. Masses are assessed for their size, shape, margins, and density. The shape may be round, oval, lobulated, or irregular. Margins are generally described as circumscribed (sharply defined) (**Fig. 2**), indistinct (**Fig. 3**), spiculated (**Fig. 4**), or microlobulated; the later three usually, but not always, are malignant masses. When all or part of the margin is abutting the normal glandular parenchyma and not amenable to precise evaluation, the term "obscured margin" is used. The density is

described as high, equal, or low relative to glandular breast parenchyma. Density of the mass is not very helpful for characterization of masses. Exception is fat-containing masses, which are always benign and are described as such (**Fig. 5**).

Calcifications are commonly encountered on mammograms and most of these are benign. Calcifications are evaluated for their number, size, shapes, distribution, and any characteristic morphology. Calcifications are broadly classified into typically benign, intermediate concern, and high probability of malignancy. Most benign calcifications are larger than 0.5 mm. Typically, benign calcifications include skin calcifications (**Fig. 6**), vascular calcifications, popcorn calcifications of involuted fibroadenoma (**Fig. 7**), eggshell or rim calcifications, long rodlike ductal calcifications, and coarse dystrophic calcifications. Solitary or clustered (five or more in 1 mL of breast tissue) microcalcifications are also benign if these are round and uniform in morphology. Breast cancers do not have fatty component and hence, similar to masses, any calcification with central lucency is always benign (see **Fig. 6**). Amorphous or indistinct calcifications are of intermediated concern. Calcifications with high probability of malignancy are smaller than 0.5 mm and are pleomorphic (varying sizes and shapes), fine linear, and branching casts and those that are more conspicuous than amorphous calcifications (**Fig. 8**). Distribution also modifies the characterization of the calcifications, which are not typically benign. Calcifications that are distributed over large area of the breast (regional) or diffusely scattered over entire or both breasts are benign, whereas those with segmental distribution confirming to a duct territory, those with linear branching pattern suggesting intraductal spread (see **Fig. 8**), and clustered fine irregular calcifications are suspicious for malignancy.

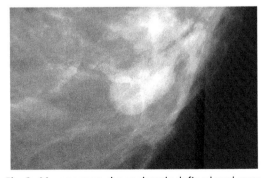

Fig. 2. Mammogram shows sharply defined oval mass, which is probably benign (BI-RADS category 3).

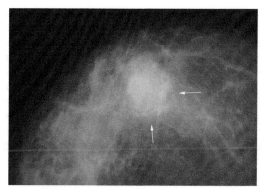

Fig. 3. Mammogram shows an oval mass with indistinct posterior margins (*arrows*), which is suspicious for cancer (BI-RADS category 4).

The term "architectural distortion" is used to describe focal distortion or tethering of the septe, focal spiculations, or the retraction of the parenchyma in absence of a mass. These may rarely represent cancer; however, most commonly these are seen as associated and not isolated findings of breast cancer (see **Fig. 1**). "Focal asymmetry" is a term used to describe the asymmetric glandular density parenchyma, which is appreciated when compared with the same area of the contralateral breast. It usually represents asymmetric but normal breast tissue; however, it must be ensured that it does not represent a mass. The focal asymmetry is suspicious if it is associated with palpable abnormality or on serial mammograms it is a new or evolving finding.[17]

MAMMOGRAPHY OF LESIONS SUSPECTED TO BE CANCER

Breast cancer may be suspected because of the palpable or imaging-detected abnormality. The

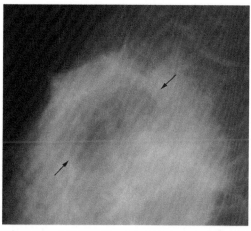

Fig. 5. A palpable mass was seen as an oval well-defined mass of fat density (*arrows*). It is a characteristic appearance of a lipoma (BI-RADS category 2).

palpable lesion may be detected by the patient herself or by the physician on clinical breast examination. Although some masses are fairly suggestive of breast cancer on clinical breast examination, others are inconspicuous, indeterminate, or have benign features on palpation. In almost all of these, an imaging evaluation is required to confirm the presence of mass; to characterize it; to search for ipsilateral multifocal (in same ductal segment or quadrant) or multicentric (distant) lesions; and to screen the contralateral breast.[18] Mammography should be performed, preferably with metallic skin marker at the site of palpable mass, because this correlates the clinical and mammographic abnormality. Failure to demonstrate the mass on mammography, however, does not rule out the presence of the lesion and biopsy is required. Similarly,

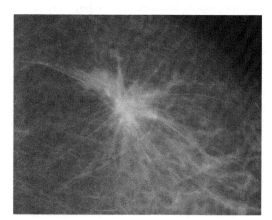

Fig. 4. Irregular spiculated mass seen on this mammogram is highly suspicious for cancer (BI-RADS category 5).

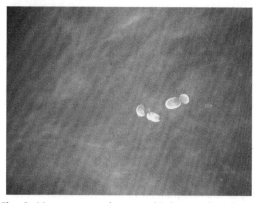

Fig. 6. Mammogram shows multiple round and oval coarse calcifications with central lucencies. These are characteristic dermal calcifications, which are benign (BI-RADS category 2).

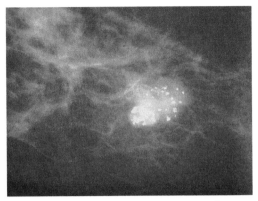

Fig. 7. Lobulated sharply defined mass with coarse calcification, some of which have a "popcorn" appearance. This is a characteristic appearance of an involuting fibroadenoma (BI-RADS category 2).

mammography cannot be used to exclude the presence of breast cancer. Mammography is a test to detect, not to diagnose, the lesion. Mammography can be diagnostic but only for few benign lesions, such as lipoma (see **Fig. 5**); hamartoma; involuting fibroadenoma with popcorn calcification (see **Fig. 7**); or small intramammary lymph nodes. Some findings, such as spiculated mass, are highly suggestive but not diagnostic of cancer (see **Fig. 4**). Postoperative scarring, fat necrosis, radial scar, and desmoids tumors can also have spiculated margin.[19] Abscesses and hematomas may also have similar appearance.

Whether palpable or not, all mammographic abnormalities must be carefully evaluated and attempt should be made to characterize these. Previous mammograms are useful to determine the significance of the questionable abnormalities, and these should also be reviewed whenever available.[20] Masses, calcifications, architectural distortions, or their combination that are not clearly benign should be systematically evaluated and BI-RADS categories assigned. If appropriate, ultrasound of the breast is important to evaluate palpation- or mammography-detected masses. If the mass is proved to be a simple cyst on ultrasound, no further work-up or follow-up is required.

BIOPSY OF SUSPECTED LESIONS

All BI-RADS 4 and 5 category lesions should be subjected to biopsy. Percutaneous large-core breast biopsies are performed using large-bore spring-loaded cutting needles or vacuum-assisted devices, and these have high accuracies. Most breast biopsies are performed under imaging guidance. Mammography (stereotactic) and ultrasound are the most commonly used guiding modalities. If the lesion is well demonstrated on ultrasound, it is preferred over stereotaxy, although selection of guiding modality for breast biopsy is generally a matter of operator preference and expertise. Most lesions are suitable for percutaneous biopsies. Previously, very small lesions (<5 mm) were not subjected to core biopsy for the fear of completely removing the lesion during biopsy. If the results are positive then the exact location of the tumor is not determined and hence therapeutic excision of the tumor site becomes difficult. Now metallic clip markers are available that can be deployed through the biopsy needle into the site of the lesion. If the biopsy result is positive and the lesion not visible on mammogram, this clip can be used for preoperative hookwire localization and surgical excision.

The biopsy results must also be correlated with mammographic features. All biopsy results that are not clearly benign or discordant with imaging or clinical features need repeat biopsy. A discordant result may represent sampling error. If the percutaneous biopsy result for a strongly suspicious mammographic lesion (BI-RADS 5) is benign, a repeat biopsy, preferably an excisional biopsy, should be undertaken to avoid missing the cancer. Most lesions with intermediate concern (BI-RADS 4) are actually benign,[21] and hence benign biopsy result is generally reliable. Regular imaging follow-up of these lesions is necessary, however, to ensure that a cancer is not missed.[22] The biopsy result reported as atypical ductal hyperplasia should also be excised because many of these lesions are then upgraded to in situ or invasive breast cancer.[23,24]

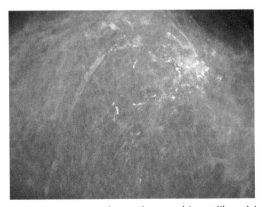

Fig. 8. Mammogram shows pleomorphic castlike calcifications, which are arranged in a linear and branching fashion conforming to the ductal distribution over wide area of the breast. It is highly suspicious for cancer (BI-RADS category 5).

PREOPERATIVE HOOKWIRE LOCALIZATION

Preoperative hookwire localization is a procedure in which a metallic hookwire is anchored in the nonpalpable breast lesion so that it can be accurately excised. The excision may be diagnostic (ie, for surgical excisional biopsy) or a therapeutic lumpectomy for breast conservation treatment (BCT). The aim of the procedure is to provide intraoperative guidance to the surgeon for accurate removal of the lesion with minimal removal of surrounding normal breast tissue and hence better cosmesis.

Many designs of the needle-hookwire assembly are available and Kopan's hookwire needle is one of the most commonly used designs. The procedure is traditionally done under mammographic guidance, but it can also be done under ultrasound or MR imaging guidance, depending on the modality on which the abnormality is demonstrated. Visibility of the lesion decides the section of the guiding modality. In mammographic procedure, open window compression paddles with alpha numeric markers are used. The area of lesion is positioned under the widow of the compression paddle and films obtained. The alpha numeric markers are visible on images and these are used to guide the needle entry. The depth of the needle is determined with orthogonal (mediolateral) view. After correct placement of the needle tip at the lesion a hookwire is introduced through the needle. The hook of the wire gets anchored in the breast just beyond the lesion. After this, the needle is withdrawn and films with wire in situ are obtained (**Fig. 9A**). The postprocedure film and in situ hookwire guides the surgeon to reach at the lesion and remove it accurately. The excised specimen is normally subjected to specimen mammography, which is performed to confirm the complete removal of the lesion in excised specimen (**Fig. 9B**). The procedure also guides the pathologist because small and marked specimens can be better evaluated and chances of the lesion missing in sectioning are minimized.[24]

With widespread use of percutaneous biopsies, such as stereotactic or ultrasound-guided core needle biopsy, this is now uncommonly performed for diagnostic reasons. Preoperative hookwire localization followed by excisional biopsy is still considered the gold standard, however, for preoperative histologic diagnosis of breast lesions.[24]

MANAGEMENT OF PROBABLY BENIGN LESIONS

The mammographic findings that normally represent benign breast lesions but unusually known to be associated with malignancy are considered probably benign (BI-RADS 3 category). Probability of malignancy in such lesions is very small, usually less than 2%, and hence routine biopsy of all such lesions is unnecessary. Instead, a short-term (normally 6 months later) follow-up mammography of the same breast is performed to determine the stability of the lesion. Any breast lesion that has any doubtful features at baseline must not be subjected to follow-up. The follow-up is aimed to prove the benign diagnosis short of biopsy and not to determine whether the lesion is benign or malignant. If the lesion is stable, the follow-up is continued usually for 2 years.[25] Any change in morphology on follow-up mammogram warrants immediate biopsy. Such lesions, even if proved malignant subsequently, do not significantly affect the stage and prognosis in most patients.[25] Indeed, many BI-RADS 3 or probably benign

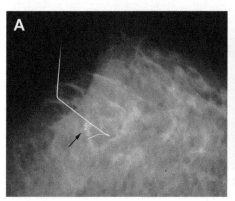
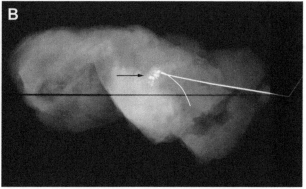

Fig. 9. (*A*) Preoperative hook wire localization. A mediolateral mammogram obtained after insertion of the hook wire and the withdrawal of the needle shows correct placement of hook wire at the clustered calcifications (*arrow*). (*B*) Postoperative specimen mammogram confirms accurate retrieval of the clustered calcifications in the excised specimen (*arrow*).

lesions are not subjected to follow-up and biopsy is undertaken because of concerns of the physician or the patient.[26,27]

PREOPERATIVE EVALUATION OF THE BREAST

After the diagnosis of breast cancer, surgery is the mainstay of the treatment. If mastectomy is planned, the role of the mammography is limited to evaluation of the contralateral breast and then its regular follow-up. BCT (wide local excision with axillary nodal clearance followed by radiotherapy) in suitable women is now a standard of breast cancer treatment and the long-term results are equivalent to mastectomies but with conservation of the breast.[28] Mammography, sometimes complimented with MR imaging, is important in patient selection for breast conservation.

The main purpose of the mammographic evaluation before BCT is to assess the extent and size of the tumor and to exclude multiple cancers. Breast cancers that are larger than 5 cm are generally not treated with BCT; however, tumor to breast size ratio is another consideration. BCT in a small-size breast with large tumor does not achieve the desired cosmesis, which is the main reason for selecting BCT over mastectomy. Size can be well assessed on mammography in most patients.

Multicentric cancer is an absolute contraindication for BCT. Multifocal tumors can be considered for BCT; however, the extent of surgical resection is wide and may not achieve the desired cosmesis (**Fig. 10**). Also, women with multiple cancers have a propensity to develop more cancers after the surgery and hence may fail the treatment.[29] The presence of suspicious calcification in and around the tumor should be carefully assessed. Clustered calcifications away from the tumor may indicate skip tumor areas. Invasive carcinoma frequently has associated component of ductal carcinoma in situ, which might extend along the ducts over a large area away from the tumor (**Fig. 11**). This is known as "extensive intraductal component." It is a frequent cause of positive margins in surgically resected specimen.[30] This requires re-exploration. Similar to the tumor size, tumor grade, and nodal status, extensive intraductal component is also considered as an important determinant of the prognosis in breast cancer. Extensive intraductal component is diagnosed on postoperative histopathology. Presence of linear branching calcification extending from the primary tumor is a strong indicator of presence of extensive intraductal component and hence this information is useful while planning the extent of surgery in BCT. Tumor may be

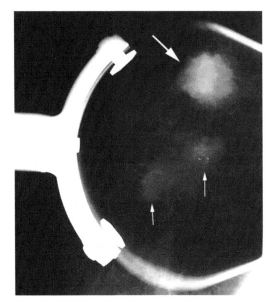

Fig. 10. Multifocal breast cancer. Spot compression mammogram of a woman with palpable breast cancer (*large arrow*) shows two additional nonpalpable smaller cancers (*small arrows*) in same quadrant of the breast.

more extensive than suspected, however, on mammography. Many ductal carcinoma in situ, especially the noncomedo type, are not always calcified and hence not appreciated on mammography.[31,32] Contralateral breast must also be carefully evaluated on mammography to detect additional cancer.

Preoperative mammographic evaluation is unsatisfactory in women with dense glandular breast.[33] Evaluation of the size and extent of the

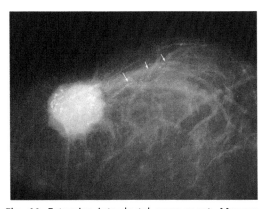

Fig. 11. Extensive intraductal component. Mammogram of a patient with palpable breast cancer shows spiculated mass with pleomorphic micro calcification. In addition, fine linear branching calcification is seen extending along the ducts from the mass toward the nipple (*arrows*).

tumor and to exclude multiple cancers is difficult in these patients. Regular posttreatment mammographic follow-up and accurate detection of recurrence is also difficult in patients with dense breasts. Breast MR imaging is superior to mammography for preoperative evaluation of both breasts[34] and has emerged as the most preferred modality for this purpose. False-positive MR imaging findings, which may result in unnecessarily extensive breast surgery or mastectomy in some patients, is an important area of concern.[35] Breast MR imaging is the most preferred modality for preoperative breast evaluation, but not yet considered mandatory. Mammography remains the basic requirement of the preoperative evaluation of breasts before BCT.

PERIOPERATIVE ASSESSMENT

Nonpalpable breast cancers undergo breast-conserving surgery with prior hookwire localization. Palpable tumors do not require this procedure. Postsurgery, the adequacy of the resection and margins can be determined on histopathology only and mammography cannot be used for this purpose. Specimen mammography is always performed if the breast cancer has calcifications. It is not always performed for masses but is useful. The specimen mammogram is performed while the patient is still on the operating table and is compared with preoperative mammogram to ensure that the abnormalities are completely included in the excised specimen. If the calcifications or mass extend to the margin of the specimen, further resection is required.[30,36] Specimen mammography is not useful if the cancer was demonstrated as an asymmetry or architectural distortion only on the preoperative mammogram.[37]

Postoperative but preradiation mammograms are valuable for postoperative assessment.[38] These may be difficult to perform and interpret in a recently operated breast. The breast is tender and adequate compression cannot be given to recently operated breasts. Postoperative hematoma and edema also makes assessment of the breast difficult and residual mass, if any, cannot be reliably excluded on mammogram. In patients who had calcifications before surgery, however, the preradiotherapy mammogram provides important information. Residual calcifications in these mammograms often, but not always, indicate residual cancer.[39] If few indeterminate calcifications are left behind but surgical margins are negative, re-excision may not be necessary.[40] If the calcifications are extensive, however, re-excision is undertaken.

NEOADJUVANT CHEMOTHERAPY

Breast cancers without distant metastases but with large tumors fixed to skin or chest wall, matted fixed axillary lymph nodes, and inflammatory breast cancers are traditionally considered as locally advanced breast cancer. Many patients with large (>5 cm) tumors are resectable but surgery may be extensive and difficult and have high chances of positive margins. These tumors are also included in locally advanced breast cancer.[41] Suitable patients with locally advanced breast cancer are treated with neoadjuvant chemotherapy with intent of downstaging the tumor. If successful, these patients are then considered for mastectomy or BCT depending on the size of the residual tumor. Patients with large tumors who desire BCT instead of mastectomy also benefit from neoadjuvant chemotherapy. Response to the neoadjuvant chemotherapy is traditionally evaluated with physical examination and mammography. After completion of the chemotherapy, residual tumor size is an important consideration for surgical planning. For this purpose, combination of mammography and ultrasound is more useful than the clinical assessment.[42] MR imaging is most accurate.[43] It is prudent to insert a metallic marker clip in these tumors before starting the neoadjuvant chemotherapy, preferably done during the biopsy. Many of these patients achieve radiologic complete response (ie, the tumor may not be visualized on mammography) (**Fig. 12**). In such situations, the metallic marker clip is then used to perform preoperative hookwire localization and local excision.[43,44] Indeed, many patients achieve pathologic complete response on

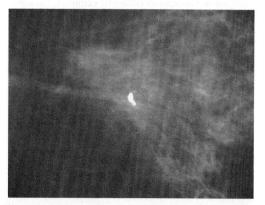

Fig. 12. Postneoadjuvant chemotherapy mammogram in a patient with locally advanced breast cancer shows near complete resolution of the mass. The marker clip seen in this mammogram can be used for preoperative localization.

neoadjuvant chemotherapy, which is proved only on postoperative histopathology.

FOLLOW-UP MAMMOGRAPHY

Patients treated with BCT need regular bilateral mammographic follow-up. It is primarily required to detect recurrence of the cancer in treated or the contralateral breast. The baseline mammogram of the treated breast is obtained at 3 to 6 months after completion of the radiotherapy. In case of tender, edematous breasts it can be delayed further. This mammogram is compared with future serial mammograms.

Several postsurgery and radiotherapy changes are apparent on follow-up mammogram after BCT. The fibrous scar develops at the operative site, which is seen as ill-defined density with adjacent architectural distortion. It may have spiculated appearance and seem suspicious (Fig. 13). Exact site of the lumpectomy must be known and review of preoperative mammograms is helpful for proper evaluation. Careful evaluation in both craniocaudal and mediolateral-oblique views is also helpful. Unlike solid mass, the scar is a two-dimensional structure formed by approximation and fibrosis of the lumpectomy cavity. Hence, size and density of the scar vary considerably in two views. Seroma is fluid collection at operative site (Fig. 14). It is usually seen as round or oval soft tissue density mass, which may persist for up to 2 years.[45] It can be ascertained by the ultrasound. Radiation changes are seen in the form of diffuse thickening of the trabeculi and the skin along with coarseness of the breast parenchyma and an overall increase in the breast density (Fig. 15). These changes are similar to the breast edema of any other cause. The severity of these changes is variable in different patients; however,

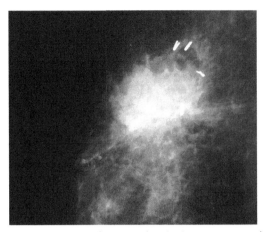

Fig. 14. Seroma at the operative site is seen as an oval ill-defined mass on this postoperative mammogram. Metallic surgical clips are also seen at the margins.

these remain stable or decrease on follow-up mammograms. Some distortion of the breast outline is also apparent after BCT and the degree depends on the extent of the excision. In addition to these changes, there may be development of calcifications in posttreatment mammograms. The causes include fat necrosis, sutural calcifications (Fig. 16), radiation induced, or dystrophic calcifications. Metallic surgical clips may also be found at the margin of the resection (see Fig. 14). These are intended to mark the lumpectomy area to which boost dose of radiation is given.

Local recurrences occur at the rate of 1% to 2% per year.[46] Although mammography is the primary modality of follow-up and detection of

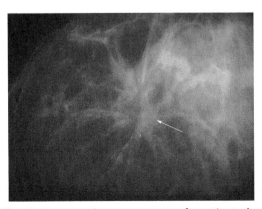

Fig. 13. Postoperative mammogram of a patient who underwent breast conservation treatment shows a spiculated scar (arrow) at operative site.

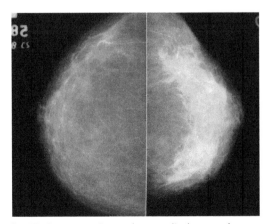

Fig. 15. Postoperative and postradiotherapy changes. Bilateral mammogram (craniocaudal views) shows increased parenchymal density, coarsening of the trabeculi, and skin thickening in the treated left breast when compared with the right breast. The left breast is also smaller in size.

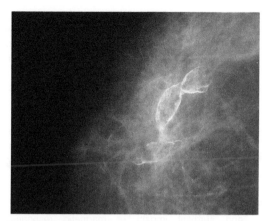

Fig. 16. Postoperative mammogram shows the characteristic appearance of sutural calcification at the operative site.

recurrences; its accuracy is lower because of distortion by the posttreatment changes. Most local recurrences are detected by mammography or by patients themselves on self-breast examination, whereas few are diagnosed on clinical breast examination.[47] The recurrences are most often seen as development of the increased density or size of the scar, new mass, or suspicious calcifications on mammography. The morphology is usually similar to that of the primary breast cancers in these patients and hence review of the preoperative mammogram is useful.[48] Enlargement or increased density of the scar or radiation changes is also suspicious.[37] MR imaging and percutaneous biopsy should be promptly obtained in case of suspicion of recurrence on mammograms.[49]

SUMMARY

Mammography is the primary imaging modality for the detection of breast cancer. Recent developments in digital mammography are expected to further improve the capabilities of this modality. Suspicious lesions on mammography must always be biopsied for the diagnosis of breast cancer. Mammography also makes important contributions in management decisions and the posttreatment follow-up of patients with breast cancer. Other imaging modalities greatly compliment, but generally do not replace, mammography.

REFERENCES

1. Elmore JG, Armstrong K, Lehman DC, et al. Screening for breast cancer. JAMA 2005;293(10): 1245–56.

2. Mushlin AI, Kouides RW, Shapiro DE. Estimating the accuracy of screening mammography: a meta-analysis. Am J Prev Med 1998;14:143–53.

3. Chiarelli AM, Majpruz V, Brown P, et al. The contribution of clinical breast examination to the accuracy of breast screening. J Natl Cancer Inst 2009;101(18): 1236–43.

4. Kopans DB. Evaluating women with lumps, thickening, discharge, or pain: imaging women with signs or symptoms that might indicate breast cancer. In: Kopans DB, editor. Breast imaging. Philadelphia: Lippincott, Williams & Wilkins; 2007. p. 733–51.

5. Mettler FA, Upton AC, Kelsey CA, et al. Benefits versus risks from mammography: a critical assessment. Cancer 1996;77:903–9.

6. D'Orsi CJ, Newell MS. Digital mammography: clinical implementation and clinical trials. Semin Roentgenol 2007;42(4):236–42.

7. Lewin JM, Hendrick RF, D'Orsi CJ, et al. Comparison of full field digital mammography with screen-film mammography for cancer detection: results of 4945 paired examinations. Radiology 2001;218:873–80.

8. Skane P, Young K, Skeinnald A. Population based mammography screening: comparison of screen-film and full field digital mammography with soft copy reading. The Oslo1 study. Radiology 2003; 229:877–80.

9. Pisano E, Gastonis C, Hendrick E, et al. Diagnostic performance of digital versus film mammography for breast cancer screening. N Engl J Med 2005; 353:1773–83.

10. Berman CG. Recent advances in breast specific imaging. Cancer Control 2007;14(4):338–49.

11. Birdwell RL, Bandodkar P, Ikeda DM. Computer aided detection with screening mammography in a university hospital setting. Radiology 2005;236: 451–7.

12. Noble M, Bruening W, Uhl S, et al. Computer aided detection mammography for breast cancer screening: systematic review and meta-analysis. Arch Gynecol Obstet 2009;279(6):881–90.

13. Poplack SA, Tosteson TD, Kogel CA, et al. Digital breast tomosynthesis: initial experience in 98 women with abnormal digital screening mammography. AJR Am J Roentgenol 2007;189:616–23.

14. Lewin IM, Isaacs PK, Vance V, et al. Dual energy contrast enhanced digital subtraction mammography: feasibility. Radiology 2003;229:261–8.

15. The ACR breast imaging reporting and data system (BI-RADS). Available at: http://www.acr.org/SecondaryMainMenusCategories/Quality Safety/BIRADSAtlas/BIRADSAtlasExcarpetedText/ BIRADSMammographyFourthEdition.aspx. Accessed September 15, 2009.

16. D'Orsi CJ, Newel MS. BI-RADS decoded: detailed guidance on potentially confusing issues. Radiol Clin North Am 2007;45:751–63.

17. Leung JWT, Sicles EA. Developing asymmetry identified on mammography: correlation with imaging outcome and pathologic findings. AJR Am J Roentgenol 2007;188:667–75.

18. Evans WP. Breast masses. Radiol Clin North Am 1995;33:1085–108.

19. Kopans DB. Suspicious lesions and lesions with high probability of malignancy. In: Kopans DB, editor. Breast imaging. Philadelphia: Lippincott Williams & Wilkins; 2007. p. 513–53.

20. Roelofs AAI, Karssemeijer N, Wedekind MS, et al. Importance of comparison of current and prior mammograms in breast cancer screening. Radiology 2007;242:70–7.

21. Oerl SG, Kay N, Reynolds C, et al. BI-RADS categorization as a predictor of malignancy. Radiology 1999;211:845–50.

22. Lee CH, Philpotts LE, Horvath LJ, et al. Follow up of breast lesions diagnosed as benign with stereotactic core needle biopsy: frequency of mammographic change and false negative rate. Radiology 1999;212:189–94.

23. Hoorntie LE, Peters PH, Mati WP, et al. Vacuum assisted breast biopsy: a critical review. Eur J Cancer 2003;39:1676–83.

24. Kopans DB. Interventional procedures in the breast: imaging guided needle placement for biopsy and the preoperative localization of clinically occult lesions. In: Kopans DB, editor. Breast imaging. Philadelphia: Lippincott Williams & Wilkins; 2007. p. 889–974.

25. Sickles E. Periodic mammographic follow-up of probably benign lesions: results in 3184 consecutive cases. Radiology 1991;179:463–8.

26. Lehman C, Holt S, Peacock S, et al. Use of the American College of Radiology BI-RADS guidelines by community radiologists. AJR Am J Roentgenol 2002;179:15–20.

27. Graf O, Helbich TH, Fuchsjaeger MH, et al. Follow-up of palpable circumscribed non calcified breast masses at mammography and US: can biopsy be averted? Radiology 2004;233(3):850–6.

28. Veronesi U, Cascinelli N, Mariani L, et al. Twenty year follow up of a randomized study comparing breast conserving surgery with radical mastectomy for early breast cancer. N Engl J Med 2002;347:1227–32.

29. Kutz JM, Jacquemier J, Amalric R, et al. Breast conserving therapy for macroscopically multiple cancers. Ann Surg 1991;212:38–44.

30. Kurniawan ED, Wong MH, Windle I, et al. Predictors of surgical margin status in breast conserving surgery within a breast screening program. Ann Surg Oncol 2008;15(9):2542–9.

31. Holland R, Hendricks J, Verbeek, et al. Extent, distribution and mammographic/histologic correlations of breast ductal carcinoma in situ. Lancet 1990;335:519–22.

32. Umetsu T, Yuen S, Kasami M, et al. Comparison of magnetic resonance imaging, multidetector row computed tomography, ultrasonography and mammography for tumor extension of breast cancer. Breast Cancer Res Treat 2008;112(3):461–74.

33. Bozzini A, Renne G, Meneghetti L, et al. Sensitivity of imaging for multifocal-multicentric breast carcinoma. BMC Cancer 2008;8:275.

34. Berg WA, Gutlerrez L, NessAlver MS, et al. Diagnostic accuracy of mammography, clinical examination, US, and MR imaging in preoperative assessment of breast cancer. Radiology 2004;233:830–49.

35. Houssami N, Ciatto S, Macaskill P, et al. Accuracy and surgical impact of magnetic resonance imaging in breast cancer staging: systematic review and meta-analysis in detection of multifocal and multicentric cancer. J Clin Oncol 2008;26(19):3248–58.

36. Schaefer FK, Eden I, Schaefer PJ, et al. Factors associated with one step surgery in case of non palpable breast cancer. Eur J Radiol 2007;64(3):426–32.

37. Dershaw DD. Breast imaging and the conservative treatment of breast cancer. Radiol Clin North Am 2002;40(3):501–16.

38. Dershaw DD. Evaluation of the breast undergoing lumpectomy and radiation therapy. Radiol Clin North Am 1995;33:1147–60.

39. Gluk BS, Dershaw DD, Liberman L, et al. Microcalcifications on post operative mammograms as an indicator of adequacy of tumor excision. Radiology 1993;188:469–72.

40. Lally BE, Haffty BG, Moran MS, et al. Management of suspicious or indeterminate calcifications and impact on local control. Cancer 2005;103:2236–40.

41. Conzen SD, Grushko TA, Olpade OI. Cancer of the breast. In: DeVita VT, Lawrence TS, Rosenberg SA, editors. DeVita, Hellman, and Rosenberg's principles and practice of oncology. 8th edition. Philadelphia: Lippincott, Williams & Wilkins; 2008. p. 1595–654.

42. Peintnger F, Kuerer HM, Anderson K, et al. Combination of mammography and sonography is useful in predicting tumor response in breast cancer patients after neoadjuvant chemotherapy. Ann Surg Oncol 2006;13(11):1443–9.

43. Yeh E, Slanetz P, Kopans DB, et al. Prospective comparison of mammography, sonography and MRI in patients undergoing neoadjuvant chemotherapy for palpable breast cancer. AJR Am J Roentgenol 2006;184:868–77.

44. Nadeem R, Chagla LS, Harris O, et al. Tumor localization with a metal coil before administration of neoadjuvant chemotherapy. Breast 2005;14:403–7.

45. Brenner RJ, Pfaff JM. Mammographic features after conservation therapy for malignant breast

disease: serial findings standardized by regression analysis. AJR Am J Roentgenol 1996;167:171–8.

46. Dewarz JA, Arriagada R, Benhamou S, et al. (for the IGR breast group). Local relapse and contralateral tumor rates in patients with breast cancer treated with conservative surgery and radiotherapy (Institut Gustave-Roussy 1970–82). Cancer 1995;765:2260–5.

47. Montgomery DA, Krupa K, Cooke TG. Follow-up in breast cancer: does routine clinical examination improve outcome? A systematic review of literature. Br J Cancer 2007;97:1632–41.

48. Gunhan-Bilgen I, Oktay A. Mammographic features of local recurrence after conserving surgery and radiation therapy: comparison with that of the primary tumor. Acta Radiol 2007;48:390–7.

49. Dao TH, Rahmount A, Campana F, et al. Tumor recurrence versus fibrosis in the irradiated breast: differentiation with dynamic gadolinium contrast enhanced MR imaging. Radiology 1993;187:751–5.

Role of Ultrasonography in Breast Cancer Imaging

Noor M. Alnaimy, MD[a],*, Nuha Khoumais, MD[b]

KEYWORDS

• Breast • Ultrasound • Cancer • Sonography

Wild and Neal[1] first described the use of ultrasound to examine the breast in 1951. Since that time, ultrasound technology has improved significantly. Now ultrasound is the most widely used and most effective adjunctive technique to mammography. Initially, ultrasound was mainly used for lesion characterization and to provide guidance for interventional procedures. Then, automated breast ultrasound was developed as a consequence of exaggerated concern about radiation risk from mammography. Several studies showed that ultrasound, at that time, failed to detect small cancers not evident on other modalities, such as mammography or even clinical breast examination. Tremendous improvements in ultrasound technology over the years, with the development of higher resolution probes, have meant improved quality of images. Breast ultrasound examinations are cheaper than examinations using MR imaging. Also, breast ultrasound poses no radiation risk during the examination. Furthermore, the breast ultrasound examination is a much more comfortable examination than examinations requiring a mammographic compression plate. However, the operator dependence of breast ultrasound, its small field of view, and the high likelihood of false-positive and false-negative findings have limited its application in breast imaging.

The current indications of breast ultrasound are[2]

Evaluation and characterization of palpable masses and other breast-related signs and/or symptoms

Evaluation of suspected or apparent abnormalities detected on other imaging studies, such as mammography or MR imaging

Initial imaging evaluation of palpable masses in women under 30 years of age and in lactating and pregnant women

Evaluation of problems associated with breast implants

Evaluation of breasts with microcalcifications and/or architectural distortion suspicious for malignancy or highly suggestive of malignancy in a setting of dense fibroglandular tissue, for detection of an underlying mass that may be obscured on the mammogram

Guidance of breast biopsy and other interventional procedures

Treatment planning for radiation therapy

Researchers are also looking at the use of intraoperative ultrasound for helping to achieve clear margins and the use of ultrasound for distinguishing recurrence from scar.

Evaluation of the axilla for occult lymph node metastasis in patients with newly diagnosed breast cancer is an area of research. The efficacy of ultrasound as a screening study for occult masses in dense fibroglandular breasts of high-risk women or of women with newly diagnosed or suspected breast cancer is also another area of research. Berg and colleagues[3] concluded that the addition of a single-screening ultrasonographic examination to mammography for women

[a] Medical Imaging Department, King Fahad Specialist Hospital, Amer Bin Thabet Street, PO Box 15215, Dammam 31444, Saudi Arabia
[b] Department of Medical Imaging, University of British Columbia, BC Cancer Agency, 600 West 10th Aveune, Vancouver, BC V57 4E6, Canada
* Corresponding author.
E-mail address: naimynoor@yahoo.com (N.M. Alnaimy).

PET Clin 4 (2009) 227–240
doi:10.1016/j.cpet.2009.10.001

at high risk of breast cancer results in increased detection of breast cancers that are predominantly small and node negative. However, it comes with a substantial risk of false-positive results. Evaluation of annual screening ultrasound is continuing in American College of Radiology Imaging Network National Breast Ultrasound Trial (ACRIN 6666) as is the evaluation of a single-screening MR imaging in these women. Breast ultrasound should be considered as a secondary evaluation or diagnostic tool rather than a routine screening modality.

Ultrasound is not appropriate

- As a substitute for mammographic screening
- For measuring response to treatment (inaccurate for sizing large tumors)
- For assessing chest wall invasion
- For assessing saline implant integrity (clinical diagnosis)
- For assessing integrity of silicone implants (better assessed by MR imaging)

PERFORMANCE OF BREAST ULTRASOUND
Transducers

Sonography of the breast basically involves production of high-frequency sound waves that penetrate the breast tissue. The waves scatter away from the transducer and are absorbed by the breast tissue, or they are reflected back to the transducer. Some of the absorbed sound can be converted in to heat as well.

Each wave scatters and attenuates as it passes through tissue. With increased tissue depth, the signal strength rapidly weakens as it bounces back to the transducer. A computer can boost the apparent decrease in signals and provide more uniform images. The computer monitor can display markers to indicate the depth of the tissue responsible for the sound reflection.

Because the sound waves are traveling parallel, the structures struck directly by those waves are seen most clearly. Images of those structures most directly in the path of the resolving power are captured in axial resolution. The lateral resolution refers to the resolution of structures on either side of the beam. The quality of this resolution is always less than that of the axial resolution. Another factor that can compromise the image quality is defocusing, which bends the sound waves as they pass through the tissue. This bending increases with increasing depth. It is strongly recommended to have broadband linear electronically focused high-frequency transducers. The center frequency should be 10 MHz, with frequency ranging as high as 17 MHz in the near field and as low as 5 MHz

deeper in the image field, thus enabling great penetration of the posterior breast tissue and pectoral muscle. For efficient survey scanning, a high-frequency broad bandwidth probe with a large footprint, such as 38 mm or even 50 mm, is useful. Small footprints, such as 18 mm, are informative in superficial lesions as well as in applications involving stand-off pads. Extended field of view or panoramic view is a helpful tool to image large lesions or to better understand relationships among multiple lesions.

Field of View

Field of view should be adjusted according to the thickness of the tissue being scanned.

Focal Zone

The focal zone should be set at the level of the lesion. Multiple focal zones can be used with the most anterior zone set at the middle of the mass. Frame rate should be 15 frames per second to maintain the benefits of real-time scanning.

Harmonics

Harmonics are used to reduce noise by cancelling the primary sound waves and allowing the passage of the first or second echo. On the basis of 254 lesions in 219 women who underwent conventional as well as harmonic imaging, Szopinski and colleagues[4] concluded that depiction of breast tissue improved with harmonics compared with conventional imaging. The use of harmonics did not change the management of any of the studied lesions.

Compound Imaging

Compound imaging has been used for many years. Among the most successful compound imaging techniques for reducing noise has been spatial compounding, in which several overlapping sound beams are angled into tissue so the central focus of a given image is clearly depicted. This technique smoothes the image and clarifies the marginal characteristics and surrounding parenchyma.

Patient Positioning

Patient positioning[4] for ultrasound scanning and for interventional procedures is one of the most important aspects of the technique. The principle is to minimize the thickness of tissue for the ultrasound beam to traverse. For lesions in the upper outer quadrant, the patient should be turned on her contralateral side with a supporting pillow/wedge placed behind her shoulder and upper back. The arm of the side being scanned should

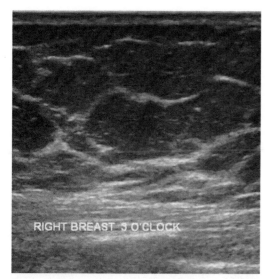

RIGHT BREAST 3 O'CLOCK

Fig. 1. Breast ultrasound in sagittal view showing different layers of parenchyma, including the underlying pectoralis muscle.

be elevated but relaxed with the wrist and hand behind the neck or near the head. For medial breast lesions, a supine position shifts the breast laterally and flattens the medial half of breast tissue, allowing adequate scanning.

SONOGRAPHIC ANATOMY OF THE BREAST

The breast anatomy, as revealed through ultrasound, is distinctive with the structural composition of the breast parenchyma varying depending on age, functional status, and parenchymal pattern, according to the individual differences in distribution and quantity of tissue. In sagittal view (**Fig. 1**), the breast contains the following structures from anterior to posterior: subcutaneous fat; cooper ligaments; the superficial mammary facia; the fibroglandular tissue, including the interlobar fibrofatty tissue; the deep mammary fascia; retromammary fat; muscle fascia; the pectoralis major and the pectoralis minor muscles; the ribs; intercostals spaces; and, lastly, pleura and lung. As a general rule, the breast tissue in young women consists mostly of parenchyma and little fat. With aging, the glandular tissue is replaced by connective tissue and fat. But the breast varies individually and, even in young girls, a substantial portion of breast may consist of fat, especially if the breast is large. These variables should be considered during breast examination as it will influence the overall interpretation of the clinical, sonographic, and mammographic findings (**Table 1**).[5,6]

DOPPLER READING IN BREAST CANCER IMAGES

The use of Doppler technology in forming breast cancer images permits two-dimensional imaging of blood flow within a real-time B-mode image. The measured frequency shifts are color-coded and displayed as color pixels (**Fig. 2**). The shade and brightness of the colors encode the direction and velocity of the flow. Such assessment can be enhanced further by activating the duplex mode. With sufficient sensitivity, the technique can detect small vessels not seen by B-mode image, which is critical in the evaluation of tumors. Dynamic examination of the breast includes spatial extension and compression.[5,6]

In a spatial extension evaluation, the breast should be examined with two-dimensional imaging techniques that cover all breast dimensions. The transducer can be angled and maneuvered to cover all mammary tissue, which is vital to assess masses and to differentiate hypoechoic tumors from normal breast tissue, such as fat lobules. Fat lobules can clearly be defined by

Table 1
Echogenicity of the breast tissue component in ultrasound

Anatomic Structure	Echogenicity
Skin	Hyperechoic
Nipple	Hypoechoic
Parenchyma	Hyperechoic
Connective tissue	Hyperechoic
Subcutaneous fat	Hypoechoic
Fatty infiltration	Hypoechoic
Retromammary fat	Hypoechoic
Cooper ligaments	Hyperechoic
Lactiferous ducts	Anechoic

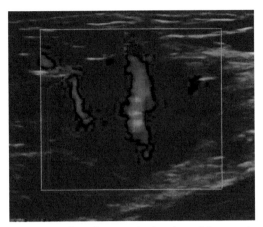

Fig. 2. Doppler ultrasound showing rich vascular tumor with malignant features.

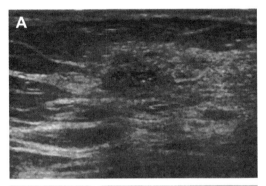

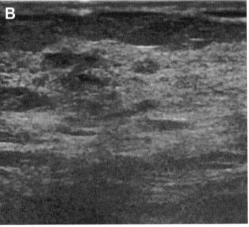

Fig. 3. Ultrasound of focal fibrocystic changes without compression (*top*) and with compression (*bottom*) showed further spreading of the parenchyma and compression.

real-time dynamic scanning and be easily distinguished by their unique spindle shape, which merges with the rest of the parenchyma at different angles and planes of imaging. By comparison, genuine tumors stand out in a discrete way with distinctive borders in all planes of imaging.[5]

With compression, another way of assessing mass in the breast, minimal pressure is applied on the breast tissue to assess the compressibility of an area of interest. Glandular tissue and fat are easily compressible while masses show variable degrees of resistance to any applied pressure. Compressibility assessment is also useful in cases where artifacts have been created by tangential beam incidence on normal connective tissue. In such cases, the pressure will flatten the parenchyma and improved sound transmission will cause artificial shadowing to fade (**Fig. 3**).

ELASTOGRAPHY

The principle of elastography is that tissue compression produces strain (displacement) within the tissue and that the strain is smaller in harder tissue than in softer tissue. Therefore, by measuring the tissue strain induced by compression, we can estimate tissue hardness, which may be useful in diagnosing breast cancer. Elastography has been used clinically to examine a variety of breast lesions in patients. This modality may be useful for differentiating malignant from benign masses. During elastography, it is assumed that the main displacement of tissue occurs in the longitudinal direction (ie, in the direction of the beam). This condition can be largely met by applying compression with a well-controlled stepping motor. With freehand compression, the

influence of probe movement on the skin's surface in the lateral direction (so-called "creep" or "slip") must be suppressed. A high-speed algorithm for estimating strain distribution is required for real-time measurement. For an elastography system to be ideal, it should have a large dynamic range of strain that does not depend on the speed and extent of compression. This would ensure stable measurements. Three methods have been introduced for measuring tissue strain in elastography. These are (1) the spatial correlation method, (2) the phase-shift tracking method, and (3) the combined auto-correlation method.[7]

The spatial correlation method uses an ordinary two-dimensional pattern-matching algorithm to search for the position that maximizes the cross-correlation between regions of interest selected from two images (one obtained before and the other obtained after deformation). This method can be used to demonstrate displacement in two dimensions (longitudinal and lateral). However, processing time is lengthy, which is a disadvantage for real-time assessment.

The phase-shift tracking method is based on an auto-correlation method well known as a principle of color Doppler ultrasonography. Because of phase-domain processing, this method can rapidly and precisely determine longitudinal tissue motion. This method poorly compensates for movement in the lateral direction, which is a disadvantage for freehand compression.

The third method, the combined auto-correlation method, enables rapid and accurate detection of longitudinal displacement by using phase-domain processing without aliasing. Because lateral and elevational tissue movements are inevitable during palpationlike freehand manipulation of the probe, elasticity images are obtained as motion images, with the patient in the supine position and with the stabilizer-equipped probe oriented perpendicular to the chest wall. The probe is applied to the breast and is moved slightly inferior and superior to obtain the elasticity images.

Approaches to elasticity imaging can be classified by the modality of the signal source (primarily ultrasound or MR imaging), by the estimated mechanical parameter (eg, stress, strain, or modulus), or by a descriptor of the experimental procedure ("dynamic" or "[quasi]static" techniques).

The mechanical properties estimated with these techniques are related. As described earlier, stress and strain are mutually responsive quantities, but they are not intrinsic material properties. Images of stress and strain are maps of a parameter relative to its surroundings (as mammogram maps the relative x-ray attenuation, for example). Elastic moduli are intrinsic material properties generally described with a matrix (as described earlier). However, in experiments under practical conditions the moduli are manipulated and their material properties (eg, incompressibility and homogeneity) are altered.

DISPLAYING, LABELING, AND MEASURING LESIONS

The lesion should be scanned in two orthogonal planes to enable adequate characterization. Perpendicular views should always be obtained. There are two different ways of measuring lesions: longitudinal and transverse. This nomenclature is appropriate if the long axis of the lesion parallels the long or short axis of the body. Radial and antiradial measurements are taken relative to the nipple with the antiradial plan orthogonal to the radial plane. Labels should identify the breast as either right or left, indicate the scan plan, and show the distance from the nipple in centimeters.

Additional information can be added (eg, palpable, tender).[2]

AUTOMATED WHOLE BREAST ULTRASOUND

Automated whole-breast ultrasound (AWBU) is a computer-based system for performing and recording ultrasound of the whole breast. The images are collected with multifrequency transducers within at least the 7- to 12-MHz range. The transducer is attached to a computer-guided mechanical arm, and images are acquired in longitudinal rows (acquiring transverse images), overlapping 7 to 10 mm to ensure complete coverage. As the transducer faces in more than 95% of the examinations measure 5.2 cm, the width of rows without overlap is about 4.2 to 4.5 cm. In most women, the number of rows varies from four to seven for each breast. The mechanical arm controls transducer speed and position, with a trained ultrasound technologist maintaining appropriate contact pressure and orientation vertical to the skin. Approximately 150 to 300 images per row are immediately displayed on the AWBU monitor and then permanently stored.

The typical imaging time is 10 to 20 minutes for each participant, with additional participant preparation times of 5 to 10 minutes. Interpretation and reporting time for an experienced radiologist is 7 to 10 minutes per examination for typical AWBU studies. AWBU software creates a cine loop of the images for interpretation, simulating the appearance of real-time imaging. Each cine loop varies from 2000 to 5000 images, depending on breast size, with about 3000 images for the average woman. Lesion detection is enhanced by review of the cine loop at about 10 images per second to simulate motion through the breast. Single still images are reviewed only after a possible abnormality has been identified. Using spatial registration recorded as images are acquired, any point on an image can be identified as a distance from the nipple in a specific radius. Images can be played back on a high-resolution monitor, enabling users to view three-dimensional reconstruction and to adjust compressed image size, contrast, brightness, and review speed.

Kevin and colleagues[8] evaluated 6425 AWBU examinations and mammograms performed on 4419 asymptomatic women. Breast cancer detections doubled from 23 to 46 in 6425 studies using AWBU with mammography, resulting in an increase in diagnostic yield from 3.6 per 1000 with mammography alone to 7.2 per 1000 by adding AWBU. Sensitivity for mammography alone was 40% but increased to 81% with the addition of AWBU. Sensitivity of AWBU alone was 67%.

Specificity is 89.9% for AWBU, 95.15% for mammography, and 98.7% for combined mammography and AWBU. The investigators concluded that AWBU with mammography is significantly better than mammography alone for detecting breast cancer, especially in dense breasts. Women with dense breasts face a particularly difficult situation, as they may be at higher risk of developing breast cancer and less likely to have the cancer detected by standard mammography screening.

The improvement in cancer detection of 3.6 per 1000 demonstrated with AWBU is similar to supplemental yield findings of earlier studies using handheld ultrasound (Range 2.7–4.6 per 1000). However, AWBU has several advantages over handheld ultrasound. First, it provides more reproducible, thorough imaging through the entire breasts. Second, it has higher definition with better contrast and sharpness and smaller images for review by using a high-resolution 2000-line reading monitor with three-dimensional capability. Third, it enables delayed interpretation at computer monitor–based reading stations with non–real-time review, optimizing the radiologist's reading environment.[8]

ULTRASOUND-GUIDED INTERVENTIONAL PROCEDURE

Ultrasound-guided interventional procedures in breast cancer are used mainly for diagnostic purposes, such as tissue sampling, whether it is fine needle aspiration biopsy or core needle biopsy. Presurgical needle localization is another major indications for the ultrasound-guided approach in interventional procedures. Ultrasound is one of several imaging techniques that may be used to guide interventional procedures. Other breast imaging modalities used for guidance include mammography (conventional and stereotactic), MR imaging, and CT.

Developers of other techniques for detecting suspicious breast lesions should concede the need for a capability to biopsy lesions that are uniquely detected by those modalities, and they should attempt to develop such a capability along with their techniques. Before the performance of any ultrasound-guided interventional procedure, the lesion should be evaluated completely with dedicated ultrasound study so that the mass or masses are evaluated with full characterization and proper categorization according to the Breast Imaging Reporting and Data System (BIRADS). Once this evaluation is completed, the target can be determined. Correlation between findings on other imaging modalities (eg, mammography or

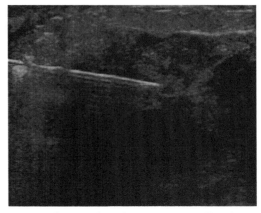

Fig. 4. Ultrasound-guided core needle biopsy showing 14-gauge needle through suspicious nodule, which proved to be invasive ductal carcinoma.

MR imaging) or on clinical examination and ultrasound should be made prior to any interventional procedure.

Indications

Indications for ultrasound-guided biopsy are as follows

- simple and complicated cysts, to facilitate aspiration and cytology
- complex and solid masses, to facilitate core needle biopsy (**Fig. 4**) or fine needle aspiration
- masses assessed as highly suggestive of malignancy (BIRADS category 5), to confirm the diagnosis and guide definitive treatment
- masses assessed as suspicious abnormalities (BIRADS category 4)
- management planning if there is more than one suspicious mass, particularly masses

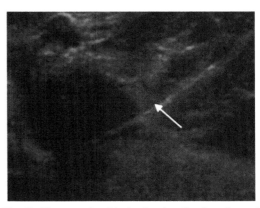

Fig. 5. Ultrasound-guided wire localization (*arrow*) for nonpalpable invasive ductal carcinoma.

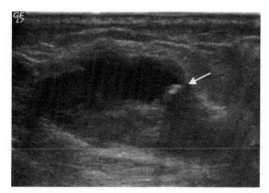

Fig. 6. Placement of coil marker (*arrow*) before chemoradiotherapy.

occupying more than one quadrant (ie, multicentric distribution)

For lesions that are probably benign (BIRADS category 3) but biopsy indicated at short-interval follow-up

For suspicious areas of enhancement appreciated on contrast-enhanced breast MR imaging and detected on "targeted" ultrasound examination correlation presurgical localization

For guide-wire localization: Ultrasound-guided wire localization is performed (**Fig. 5**) when the lesion is shown in ultrasound, but is not detected clinically or by palpation. In such a case, dedicated ultrasound with comprehensive evaluation is performed and, after the malignancy is confirmed by biopsy, the targeted mass is localized under

---

Box 1
Individual sonographic characteristics

Malignant[a]

Nonparallel

Angular margins

Shadowing

Branch pattern

Hypoechogenicity

Calcification

Duct extension

Microlobulation

Benign[b]

Absent malignant findings

Intense hyperechogenicity

Elliptical shape

Gentle bi/trilobulations

Thin, echogenic pseudocapsule

Indeterminate

Maximum diameter

Isoechogenicity

Mild hypoechoenicity

Normal/enhanced sound transmission

Hetero/homogenous echotexture

[a] If even a single malignant feature is present, the nodule is excluded from benign classification.
[b] Individual benign features for a nodule to be classified as benign. However, combinations of findings could result in a benign classification: (1) intense and uniform hyperechogenicity, (2) elliptical shape and thin echogenic capsule, (3) two or three gentle lobules with thin echogenic capsule

Table 2
Benign sonographic characteristics versus benign histologic findings

Characteristic	Sensitivity	Specificity
Hyperechogenicity	100%	7.4%
Two or three lobulations	99.2%	19.4%
Elliptical shape	97.6%	51.2%
Thin capsule	95.2%	76.0%

guidance of real-time ultrasound and the wire is placed within the tumor core, with the free end of the wire fixed to the skin and secured by adhesive band. The approach to the target lesion depends on its location. For instance, lesions on outer quadrants are approached laterally.

positioning a marking device: During ultrasound-guided biopsy, a marker (**Fig. 6**) can be placed within the biopsied tumor to localize the mass after therapy. The markers come in different shapes and some are used in MR image–guided procedures as well. In ultrasound, the marker appears echogenic and exhibits posterior shadowing

biopsy of lymph nodes in the axilla or intramammary lymph node at the axillary tail in cases of known or suspected malignancy

If breast imaging shows findings that lead to suspicion of malignancy, and if abnormal lymph nodes are seen within the axilla or axillary tail, fine needle aspiration or core biopsy sampling of the cortex of the abnormal lymph node can be performed at the time of initial imaging-guided core biopsy of the suspicious breast mass, or at a later time. Another indication for lymph node biopsy is failure of imaging modalities to detect a mass within the breast despite the existence of a suspicious lymph node.

Special care should be taken if the core biopsy is performed in the axilla because of the presence of sensitive structures (the brachial plexus and axillary artery and vein)

Repeat ultrasound-guided percutaneous core or vacuum-assisted needle biopsy sampling is an alternative to surgical biopsy when the initial core biopsy results are nondiagnostic or discordant with the imaging findings, or if an initial fine needle aspiration biopsy yields atypical, suspicious, or nondiagnostic cytology

Contraindications

An important contraindication for ultrasound-guided biopsy is failure to visualize the target or breast lesion sonographically. Before the procedure, potential bleeding stemming from a history of a bleeding diathesis, allergies, and use of such medications as aspirin or anticoagulants should be dealt with in a watchful way.[9]

EVALUATION OF BREAST LUMPS AND MASSES
Palpable Mass with Benign Clinical Impression

Ultrasound features of a benign breast lesions
The accuracy of breast ultrasound in characterization of breast cyst approaches 100%. According to sonographic criteria, simple cysts are circumscribed round, oval, or gently lobulated, anechoic masses, with posterior enhancement. These findings in a simple cyst are suggestive of benign pathology (BIRADS category 2). Ultrasound-guided cyst aspiration can be performed if the patient is symptomatic with pain or if a very large cyst was documented. Cloudy yellow, greenish, and black aspirate are typical of benign cyst

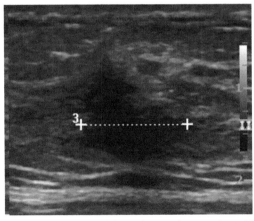

Fig. 7. Malignant nodule with angular margins with spicules and posterior shadowing.

Table 3
Malignant sonographic characteristics versus malignant histologic findings

Characteristic	Sensitivity	Specificity	Accuracy
Spiculation	36%	99.4%	88.8%
Nonparallel	41.6%	8.1%	88.7%
Angular margins	83.2%	92.0%	90.5%
Shadowing	48.8%	94.7%	87.1%
Branch pattern	29.6%	96.6%	85.5%
Hypoechogenicity	68.8%	90.1%	87.2%
Calcification	27.2%	96.3%	84.8%
Duct extension	24.8%	95.2%	79.3%
Microlobulation	75.2%	83.8%	82.4%

aspirate. Smith and colleagues,[10] in their series of 660 aspirates, and Hindle and colleagues,[11] in an analysis of 689 medical records, suggest discarding the fluid unless it is bloody. It may be sent to cytology at patient request or if there is a personal history of breast cancer or atypical lesion, though there is a potential risk of false positives and atypia. It has been suggested that cysts that recur carry a potential risk of malignancy. Cysts with proliferative apocrine lining are at higher risk of recurrence and they carry a potential risk of malignancy. Complicated cysts are round or oval well-defined masses with low-level internal echoes throughout that otherwise meet the diagnostic criteria of a simple cyst. Cysts with fluid-debris levels without solid component are also considered complicated cysts. Venta and colleagues[12] found only 1 of 308 (0.3%) complicated cysts to be malignant. Neither Kolb and colleagues[13] nor Buchberger and colleagues[14] had malignancy confirmed in their series of 132 and 127, respectively. Incidental complicated cysts are classified as probably benign (BIRADS category 3). In such patients, 6-month follow up is recommended. In the context of multiple, bilateral simple cysts and a nonpalpable complicated cyst, it may be appropriate to dismiss the complicated cyst as a benign finding, though further validation of this is still ongoing. Abscesses can look like complicated cysts. They account for 16% of complicated cyst in one series. If the diagnosis of abscess is suspected clinically, on imaging, or on aspiration of fluid, the fluid should be sent for culture, a Gram stain should be ordered, and a course of antibiotics appropriate for skin organisms should be initiated. Other differential diagnoses of complicated cysts includes hematomas, fat necrosis, and galactoceles. Management should be predicated on patient symptoms.

Very small simple cysts (<4–5 mm) may appear to be solid masses or complicated cysts. They may appear indeterminate and merit aspiration and possible biopsy if solid. Oval or gently lobulated circumscribed masses with posterior acoustic enhancement or no posterior features, which might be small cysts, should be classified as probably benign. A 6-month follow-up is indicated. Clustered microcysts with thin (0.5 mm) septation are often due to apocrine metaplasia or other fibrocystic changes. They may be considered probably benign or even benign if incidental. Complex cystic masses are those with thick septation (>0.5 mm), thick wall, intracystic mass, or otherwise mixed cystic and solid components. These are suspicious for malignancy (23%). Other

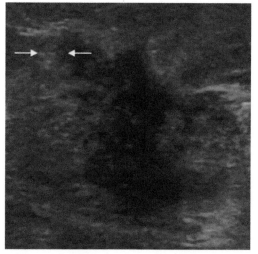

Fig. 8. Ultrasound demonstrating nonparallel hypoechoic nodule with thick ill-defined echogenic border (*between arrows*).

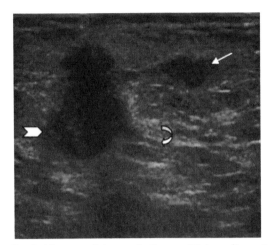

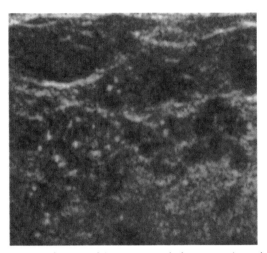

Fig. 9. Ultrasound demonstrating multiple malignant features, including angular margins (*arrowhead*), duct extension (*arrow*), branching pattern (*curved arrow*) and posterior acoustic shadowing.

Fig. 11. Ultrasound images revealed nonmarginated hypoechoic parenchymal changes with multiple echogenic foci in keeping with clustered microcalcification.

benign lesions include lipomas, lymph nodes, and fibroadenomas. Probably benign lesions have been defined by Stavros as lesions that lack malignant features (spiculations, angular margins, marked hypoechoginicity, shadowing, calcifications, duct extension, branch pattern, or microlobulation) (**Box 1**).[15] To be classified as benign, lesions should be uniformly hyperechoic, have oval shape with thin echogenic pseudocapsule, or have two or three gentle lobulations with an echogenic pseudocapsule. These have more than 98% chance of being benign (fibroadenoma) (ie, the chance of malignancy is <2%) (**Table 2**).

Ultrasound features of malignant breast lesions

Breast cancer is heterogeneous. The malignant breast nodule is not entirely composed of tumor cells. In many cases, the nodule is also composed of extracellular matrix and host reaction. All three components contribute to the sonographic appearance, gross morphologic findings, and histologic findings. The heterogeneous population of breast cancers can present itself as circumscribed, spiculated (**Fig. 7**), or mixed circumscribed and spiculated masses. Most circumscribed carcinomas are high-grade invasive duct carcinomas or medullary, colloid, and invasive papillary carcinomas. Spiculated masses are usually low- to

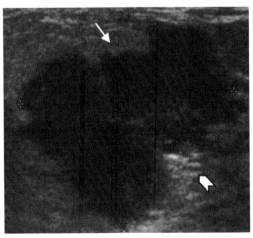

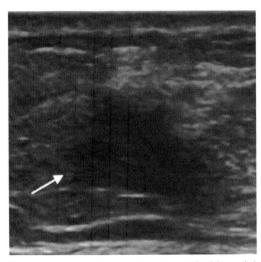

Fig. 10. Ultrasound of nonparallel hypoechoic nodule with angular margins, microlobulation (*arrow*) and enhanced through transmission (*arrowhead*).

Fig. 12. Ultrasound images of tender palpable nodule showing angular margins (*arrow*), hypoechoic texture, and nonparallel alignment.

intermediate-grade invasive duct carcinomas, invasive lobular carcinomas, or tubular carcinomas. The sonographic features (**Table 3**) suspicious for malignancy can be placed into three categories: (1) surface characteristics, (2) shape, and (3) internal characteristics. Stavros and colleagues have further classified the suspicious sonographic features into hard, soft, and mixed.[15]

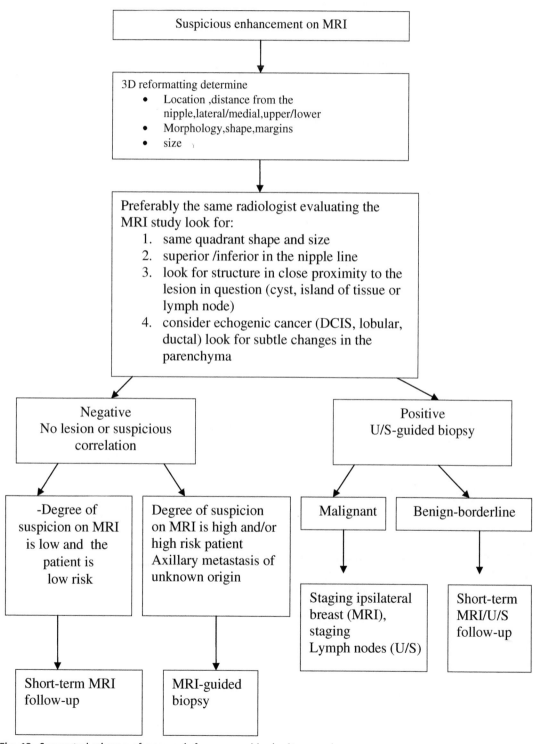

Fig. 13. Suggested scheme of approach for a second-look ultrasound.

The hard findings are suggestive of invasion. The soft findings tend to represent the ductal carcinoma-in-situ (DCIS) component of the lesion. Hard suspicious findings include angular margins (see **Figs. 7** and **8**), frank spiculation, thick ill-defined hyperechoic halo, and retrotumoral acoustic shadowing. Angular margins represent the suspicious finding that has the best combination of sensitivity and positive predictive value. The angles can be acute, obtuse, or right. They occur at the area of least resistance to invasion. Spiculations (**Figs. 9–11**) range in size from coarse to fine. The fine spiculations may not be preserved sonographically. Coarse spiculations have alternating hypo- and hyperechoic components. The hypoechoic component represents either fingers of invasive tumor or DCIS component of tumor growing into the surrounding tissue. The hyperechoic element represents the interface between the tumor and the surrounding breast tissue. Only 35% of malignant breast nodules have demonstrable frank spiculations. Hyperechoic halo (see **Fig. 8**) may represent fine spiculations that underwent volume averaging. It is typically thicker along the sides of the nodule than on the front or back of the nodule. Peritumoral inflammatory and/or angiogenic edema that occurs with high-grade invasive duct carcinomas and medullary carcinoma can also cause a thick hyperechoic halo. Lymphedema can be caused from lymphatic invasion and obstruction. Retrotumoral shadowing is a suspicious finding unique to sonography. It is more prominent in tumors with abundant desmoplasia.

Differential diagnosis for acoustic shadowing includes low- to intermediate-grade invasive duct carcinomas, invasive lobular carcinomas, and tubular carcinomas. Differential diagnosis for

enhanced sound transmission (**Fig. 12**) includes high-grade invasive duct carcinoma, colloid carcinoma (>1.5 cm in diameter), high-grade DCIS, medullary carcinoma, and invasive papillary carcinoma.

SECOND-LOOK ULTRASOUND

Second-look ultrasound, postdiagnostic breast MR imaging seems to show great promise, especially in patients who have familial or genetic predisposition to breast cancer and those suspected of having an occult carcinoma of the breast with clinically proven axillary lymph node metastasis. In a study by Sim and colleagues,[16] sonography was performed as part of a targeted examination to identify lesions also identified by MR imaging. A sonographic correlate was found in 67% of cases. Investigators concluded that second-look sonography is a user-friendly, less time-consuming alternative to MR-guided biopsy in women with familial or genetic predisposition to breast cancer. In a recent study by McMahon and colleagues,[17] both mammography and sonography were performed before MR imaging. Second-look ultrasound was able to identify 78% of the breast tumors missed on the first-look ultrasound. In patients who had axillary metastasis and no breast tumor identified on mammography and clinical examination, it may make sense to perform sonography before MR imaging. Sonography may reveal a mammographically and clinically occult malignant lesion and thus obviate MR imaging (**Fig. 14**).

If mammography and sonography are interpreted as negative or unavailable, it is important to perform three-dimensional reformatting and to

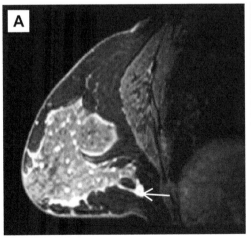
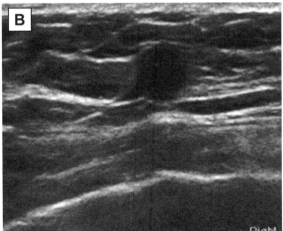

Fig. 14. (*A*) Sagittal reformatted T1-weighted image with a suspicious lesion inferiorly in the right breast (*arrow*). The lesion was missed at the time of first-look ultrasound. (*B*) The second-look ultrasound where an ill-defined round mass was identified. Histology: invasive ductal carcinoma.

obtain maximum intensity projection images of the fat-suppressed dynamic MR imaging data. The dimensions of the MR-detected lesion should be analyzed carefully. The radiologist should be mindful of the differential diagnostic possibilities based on the MR imaging. The distance from the nipple and the skin to the lesion, the quadrant or the clock-face location of the lesion, and any distinct cystic structures close to the lesion and identifiable with sonography should be noted. The distance from the nipple and the craniocaudal location with reference to the nipple is the most reliable datum. Because the patient is positioned prone for MR imaging and supine for sonography, the lesion may project in different locations on each study. Also, slight compression applied to immobilize the breast during MR imaging may affect the measurement of the distance from the skin. It is suggested that having sonography performed by the same radiologist who interpreted the MR imaging study may increase the sensitivity of targeted sonography. When a lesion cannot be identified on second-look ultrasound, clinicians should review the indication for performing the MR imaging study in the first place and the lesion's degree of suspicion for breast cancer. Current data suggest that low-risk patients more commonly have benign lesions and that benign lesions are less likely to be visualized by targeted sonography.[18,19] Therefore, it is recommended to closely follow up those patients with no sonographic correlates. Lesions detected in patients with documented metastatic adenocarcinoma in the axillary lymph nodes from an unknown primary and in those who have familial predisposition to breast cancer should be regarded with more suspicion and subjected to MR imaging–guided biopsy. When sonography-guided biopsy reveals a borderline or high-risk lesion, the clinician, the radiologist, and the pathologist should arrive at a consensus regarding management. If the management recommendations are unclear or controversial, excision should be considered because the current understanding of the natural history of lesions initially discovered on MR imaging is limited (see **Figs. 13** and **14**)

SUMMARY

Familiarity with breast ultrasound in terms of technique, indications, anatomy, and interpretation is vital for proper breast examinations. Ultrasound is a integral method of approaching breast masses and an important tool in interventional breast procedures. Combination of mammogram and ultrasound examinations when indicated is an effective method in increasing rate of cancer detection. Second-look ultrasound is an effective method to localize lesions missed in the initial scanning.

REFERENCES

1. Smith D. Breast Ultrasound. Rad Clin of N America 2001;39(3):485–97.
2. ACR practice guideline for the performance of breast ultrasound examination, 2007. Available at: www.ACR.org.
3. Berg WA, Blume JD, Cormack JB, et al. Combined screening with ultrasound and mammography vs mammography alone in women at elevated risk of breast cancer. JAMA 2008;299(18):2151–63.
4. Szopinski KT, Pajk AM, Wysocki M, et al. Tissue harmonic imaging: utility in breast sonography. J Ultrasound Med 2003;22(5):479–87.
5. Madjar H, Mendelson EB, Jellins J. The practice of breast ultrasound: techniques, findings, differential diagnosis 2008. 268 pages. Available at: http://www.books.google.com.
6. Kopans DB. Breast imaging, 2007. p. 555–7.
7. Itoh A, Ueno E, Tohno E, et al. Breast disease: clinical application of US elastography for diagnosis. Radiology 2006;239(2):341–50.
8. Kelly KM, Dean J, Comulada WS, et al. Breast cancer detection using automated whole breast ultrasound and mammography in radiographically dense breasts. Eur Radiol 2009 Sep 2 [Epub ahead of print].
9. ACR practice guideline for the performance of ultrasound-guided percutanous breast interventional procedures, 2009. Available at: www.ACR.org.
10. Smith DN, Kaelin CM, Korbin CD, et al. Impalpable breast cysts: utility of cytologic examination of fluid obtained with radiological guided aspiration. Radiology 1997;204:149–51.
11. Hindle WH, Arias RD, Florentine B, et al. Lack of utility in clinical practice of cytologic examination of non bloody cyst fluid from non palpable breast cysts. Am J obstet Gynecol 2000;182:1300–5.
12. Venta LA, Kim JP, Pelloski CE, et al. Management of complex breast cysts. AJR Am J Roentgenol 1999;173:1331–6.
13. Kolb TM, Lichy J, Newhouse JH. Occult cancer in women with dense breast: detection with screening US-diagnostic yield and tumor characteristics. Radiology 1998;207:191–9.
14. Buchberger W, Dekoekkoek-Doll P, Springer P, et al. Incidental findings on sonography of the breast: clinical significance and diagnostic work up. AJR Am J Roentgenol 1999;173:921–7.
15. Stavros AT, Rapp CL, Kaske TI, et al. Hard and soft sonographic findings of malignancy. Breast imaging: RSNA categorical course in diagnostic radiology 2005;125–42.

16. Sim LS, Hendriks JH, Bult P, et al. US correlation for MRI-detected breast lesions in women with familial risk of breast cancer. Clin Radiol 2005; 60(7):801–6.

17. McMahon K, Medoro L, Kennedy D. Breast magnetic resonance imaging: an essential role in malignant axillary lymphadenopathy of unknown origin. Australas Radiol 2005;49(5):382–9.

18. Krige M, Brekelmans CT, Boetes C, et al. Efficacy of MRI and mammography for breast cancer screening in women with familial or genetic predisposion. N Engl J Med 2004;351(5):427–37.

19. La Trenta LR, Menell JH, Morris EA, et al. Breast lesions detected with MR imaging: utility and histopathologic importance of identification with US. Radiology 2003;227(3):856–61.

Evolving Role of MRI in Breast Cancer Imaging

Susan Weinstein, MD

KEYWORDS

- Breast MRI • Breast cancer diagnosis
- Screening • Mammography

Breast cancer is the most common solid tumor diagnosed in women. The American Cancer Society estimates that there will be 192,000 new cases of breast cancer diagnosed in 2009.[1] However, mortality from breast cancer has been decreasing since the late 1980s.[1] The decreased mortality is thought to be due to multiple factors, including improved treatment regimen, and is also attributable to early detection from screening, improved diagnostic tools, and new techniques that have evolved in biopsy and breast imaging.

Mammography has been the mainstay of breast cancer screening leading to early diagnosis and improved survival. Before the advent of mammographic screening, ductal carcinoma in situ (DCIS) represented 2% of breast cancers; post mammography, DCIS composes approximately 20% of the breast cancers diagnosed. There are, however, limitations to x-ray mammography. The overall sensitivity of mammography is approximately 85%.[2] However, sensitivity can vary depending on breast density. In the fatty breast, the sensitivity of mammography has been reported to be more than 95%, but in the dense breast, sensitivity is reported to be approximately 50%[3,4] and it is reported to be even lower in BRCA1/2 mutation carriers.[5] Because there are inherent limitations in x-ray mammography, effort has been made to develop adjunctive imaging tools.

One such tool is the breast magnetic resonance imaging (MRI). The use of contrast in breast MRI to detect cancer was first reported in 1989.[6,7] Since the initial published reports, the use of breast MRI has gained wide acceptance. Today, breast MRI is widely used in many clinical applications. In patients with known breast cancer, breast MRI is used to assess for the extent of tumors, including chest wall invasion, and to assess for multifocal or multicentric tumors in the ipsilateral breast, where breast conservation therapy (BCT) is contraindicated. As simultaneous imaging of the contralateral breast is possible, the contralateral breast may be screened for clinically and mammographically occult cancer. The topic of contralateral screening is addressed in a separate article elsewhere in this issue. Other indications for breast MRI include screening of women who have greater than 20% to 25% lifetime risk for breast cancer, evaluation of clinically significant nipple discharge, additional evaluation of mammographic abnormality, monitoring response to neoadjuvant chemotherapy in patients with advanced breast cancer, and evaluation of patients who present with axillary lymph node metastasis from an occult primary.

With the use of intravenous contrast, such as gadolinium-diethylenetriamine pentaacetic acid (Gd-DTPaA), the sensitivity of MRI for invasive breast cancer approaches 100%. Without contrast, the ability to differentiate tumor from the surrounding tissue is limited. Neovascularization by the cancer serves as the basis for breast cancer imaging (**Fig. 1**). Neovascularity results in abnormal or leaky capillaries that cause rapid uptake of contrast leading to early enhancement and early wash out of contrast from the cancer, a characteristic enhancement pattern seen in many malignancies. In patients with significant background or physiologic enhancement, the

Department of Radiology, Division of Breast Imaging, University of Pennsylvania Medical Center, 3400 Spruce Street, 1 Silverstein Building, Philadelphia, PA 19104, USA
E-mail address: susan.weinstein@uphs.upenn.edu

PET Clin 4 (2009) 241–253
doi:10.1016/j.cpet.2009.09.003

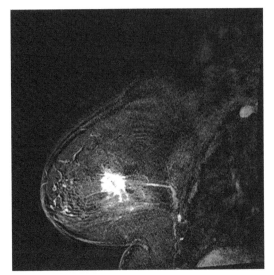

Fig. 1. A 75-year-old patient with a recent diagnosis of invasive lobular carcinoma detected on mammography. MRI demonstrates an irregular, avidly enhancing mass with washout in the lateral breast. The MRI was obtained by the surgeon before surgery to evaluate for disease extent.

background enhancement may limit the sensitivity of MRI. The degree of background enhancement, quantified as the volume and the intensity of enhancing glandular tissue, is categorized as minimal (< 25% volumetric enhancement) (Fig. 2A), mild (25%–50% volumetric enhancement), moderate (50%–75% volumetric enhancement) (see Fig. 2B), or marked (>75% volumetric enhancement) (see Fig. 2C). To minimize physiologic enhancement, it is recommended that women be imaged between day 7 and day 14 of the menstrual cycle. Although this may be possible in patients who are being screened for breast

cancer, it may not always be feasible in patients who have been recently diagnosed with breast cancer.

Although the sensitivity of breast MRI approaches 100% for invasive cancer, the specificity is lower as many benign lesions such as lymph nodes, fibroadenomas, papillomas, fat necrosis, or benign breast tissue, may enhance (Figs. 3–5). At times, it may be difficult to differentiate these benign lesions from malignancies. Although the sensitivity of MRI has been reported to be high, in the range of 71% to 100%,[8] the specificity of MRI has been variable. Prospective and retrospective screening studies have reported that the positive predictive value (PPV) of magnetic resonance (MR) biopsies ranges from 17% to 89%.[3,9–16] Sensitivity for DCIS also seems variable. There are reports that MRI is highly sensitive in detecting high-gradeDCIS, although it is less sensitive in detecting low-grade DCIS. Kuhl and colleagues[17] evaluated 167 patients with DCIS over a 5-year period. Forty-three percent (n = 72) of these patients were detected only on MRI. Of the patients detected only on MRI, 60% had high-grade DCIS, whereas approximately a third of the patients detected only through mammographs presented low-grade DCIS.

IMAGING IN PATIENTS WITH BREAST CANCER
Estimating the Extent of Disease

The most common indication for MRI is for the patient with a recent diagnosis of breast cancer. Many studies have shown that MRI can detect mammographically and clinically occult cancer.[18–25] Plans for breast conservation therapy may be changed to mastectomy based on MRI findings.

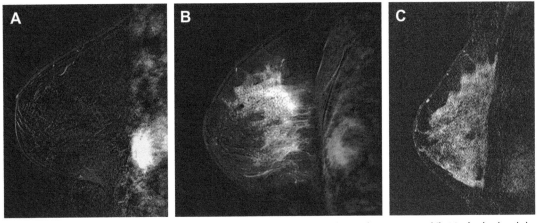

Fig. 2. (A) Minimal glandular enhancement. (B) Moderate glandular enhancement. (C) Marked glandular enhancement.

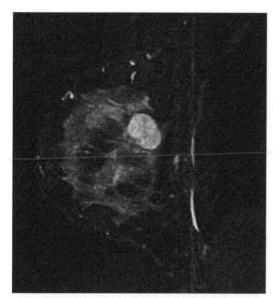

Fig. 3. There is a well-circumscribed lobulated mass in the posterior breast with nonenhancing septations. Kinetics evaluation showed progressive enhancement. The imaging findings are in keeping with a fibroadenoma.

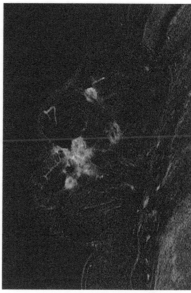

Fig. 5. A 69-year-old woman with a history of breast conservation therapy. MRI shows an irregular mass in the central breast with adjacent smaller areas of enhancement. Biopsy revealed fat necrosis.

Before changing surgical plans, the suspicious findings should be confirmed with pathology results.

Over the years, the trend for the surgical treatment of breast cancer has been toward less-invasive surgery. Halsted first described radical mastectomy, a debilitating surgery involving en bloc resection of the breast, pectoralis muscle, and axillary contents. The trend toward less-invasive

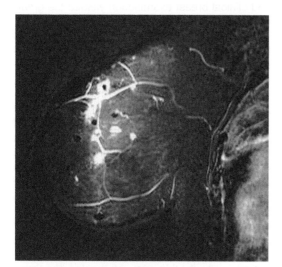

Fig. 4. Patient with multiple irregular areas of enhancement predominantly in the superior breast. MRI-guided core needle biopsy showed fat necrosis.

surgery has resulted in the acceptance of BCT. Randomized controlled studies have shown similar survival rates in patients who underwent BCT when compared with those who chose mastectomy.[26–29] The reported recurrence rates after BCT has been reported to be approximately 10%, although newer studies show a slightly lower rate.[30] It is thought that early recurrences are caused by residual disease not eradicated by adjuvant therapy, whereas the late recurrences may be due to second primaries. MRI has the potential to detect unsuspected, multicentric, and multifocal disease that could result in failure of BCT.

Studies have shown that breast MRI is able to detect multicentric, multifocal disease in 12% to 88% of patients.[31–35] The presence of additional foci of carcinoma in mastectomy specimens, separate from the primary cancer, has previously been reported and has been used as an argument against BCT. [36–38] Radiation therapy can treat some of the residual disease, and studies have shown that without radiation therapy, the failure rate can be as high as 40%.[39–41] These data support the clinical significance of the additional foci of disease. Radiation can treat small residual foci, however, the average size and grade of cancers detected on MRI have been shown to be similar to mammographically detected cancers (Fig. 6).[19] In the IBMC (International Breast MRI Consortium) 6883 study, more than half of the

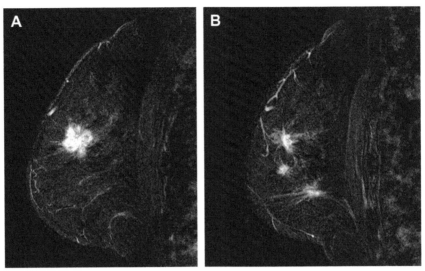

Fig. 6. Patient presented with a palpable breast mass (A). Core needle biopsy under ultrasound yielded invasive ductal carcinoma. An MRI obtained before surgery showed additional suspicious masses in the ipsilateral breast (B). Biopsy of one of the additional sites demonstrated invasive ductal carcinoma. The patient underwent mastectomy.

cancers detected on MRI measured more than 1 cm, a size that is too large to be adequately treated with radiation alone.[19]

In addition to evaluating for multicentric, multifocal cancer, MRI can better estimate tumor extent thus allowing for appropriate surgical planning and minimizing the number of surgeries. In patients who are diagnosed with breast cancer by percutaneous biopsy, a preoperative MRI may help map out the extent of disease before definitive surgery. Bedrosian and colleagues[42] studied 267 patients with known cancer. All patients had a complete conventional imaging evaluation. The patients then had MRI evaluation before definitive surgery. In 69 patients, the MRI evaluations revealed suspicious findings requiring wider surgical excision (n = 11) or excisional biopsy of a site separate from the known cancer (n = 14). In addition, 44 patients who were thought to be candidates for breast conservation therapy based on conventional imaging were converted to mastectomy based on findings seen only on MRI. Pathology results confirmed malignancy in 49 of 69 patients (71%). A suspicious area seen on MRI may be sampled using an MRI-compatible core biopsy system, and depending on the pathology result, appropriate surgical therapy may be planned for either breast conservation or mastectomy (**Fig. 7**).

Berg and colleagues[22] assessed the diagnostic accuracy of clinical breast examination, mammography, whole breast sonography, and MRI in estimating tumor extent in 111 patients with known breast cancer. The authors found ultrasound and

MRI to be more sensitive in the evaluation for invasive cancer, especially in patients with dense breasts. But no one modality detected all 177 malignancies. The addition of whole breast sonography to clinical breast examination and mammography detected additional cancers, changing surgical management in 17 of 96 patients. Subsequent use of MRI detected additional suspicious findings in 29 of 96 patients. The authors found that the addition of sonography after MRI examination did not reveal additional cancers. In the study, the combination of mammography, MRI, and clinical breast examination yielded the greatest sensitivity, with detection of all 177 cancers.

In patients with positive margins after excisional biopsy, breast MRI can assess how much residual disease is present before returning to the operating room. A postbiopsy mammogram, however, is still necessary to evaluate for residual calcifications in cases of mammographically detected DCIS. Although there are reports of DCIS detected on MRI, a negative MRI does not exclude DCIS. Depending on the extent of the disease as seen on the preoperative MRI, the surgeon could plan an appropriate surgical procedure and minimize the number of trips to the operating room. In patients with positive surgical margins, a postbiopsy MRI may be performed shortly after surgery. Although there is some compression during the MRI study, patients tolerate the examination well. A thin rim of benign-appearing enhancement may be seen around the biopsy cavity (**Fig. 8**). When there is granulation tissue,

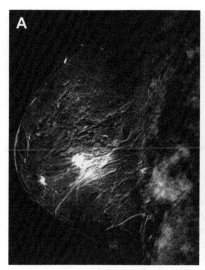 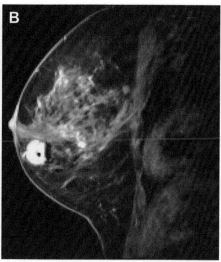

Fig. 7. A 70-year-old woman with a recent diagnosis of left breast cancer. The known cancer is located in the posterior breast. The mammogram did not reveal any additional lesions. An MRI obtained before surgery. A sub-centimeter mass was seen in the anterior breast (*A*). An MRI-guided core needle biopsy was performed (*B*). Post-biopsy changes are evident. A fluid-fluid level is present at the biopsy site. Pathology revealed in situ and invasive carcinoma. The patient was subsequently treated with mastectomy.

mild nodular enhancement may be seen. It may be difficult to differentiate between enhancing granulation tissue and residual tumor. In both situations, correlation with surgical margins can evaluate for microscopic disease that cannot be detected on MRI. The presence of thick nodular, asymmetric, bulky enhancement and its extent should be reported as suspicious for residual disease.

At the time of the MRI evaluation, assessment for chest wall invasion may be made. Both mammography and sonography have limitations in the evaluation of chest wall invasion. Chest wall invasion may also be difficult to determine on clinical assessment. Although there are limited data on MRI assessment for chest wall invasion, the obliteration of the fat plane and enhancement of the pectoralis muscle[43,44] can be indicative of muscle invasion (**Fig. 9**). Morris and colleagues[43] retrospectively reviewed MRI examinations with pathologic correlation in 19 patients with posterior breast masses. In 5 patients, MRI revealed obliteration of the fat plane with muscle enhancement; at pathologic evaluation there was chest wall invasion in all the 5 patients. When there was loss of the fat plane alone (n = 14), no chest wall invasion was present. Kazama and colleagues[44] prospectively evaluated chest wall invasion in 33 patients. Enhancement of the pectoralis muscle and loss of the fat plane were present in 7 patients. At surgery, 5 of these patients had chest wall invasion. There were 2 false positives. In the remaining 26 cases without muscle enhancement, there was no chest wall invasion on pathologic evaluation.

Patients on Neoadjuvant Therapy

In patients with inoperable locally advanced breast cancer, neoadjuvant therapy is necessary before definitive surgery. Chemotherapy is given to shrink the tumor so that surgery is feasible. Neoadjuvant therapy may also be administered for operable

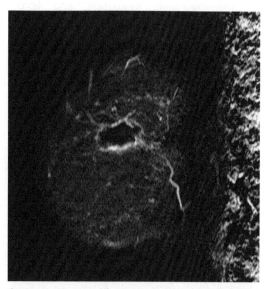

Fig. 8. A 45-year-old woman who underwent excisional biopsy for invasive lobular carcinoma. The MRI obtained postlumpectomy shows a seroma with a thin rim of enhancement with no suspicious features. The patient subsequently underwent lumpectomy and radiation therapy.

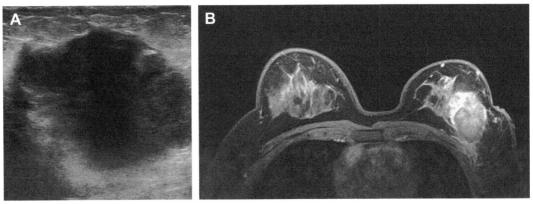

Fig. 9. A 27-year-old woman who presented with a palpable breast mass. Ultrasound evaluation of the palpable mass was initially performed revealing a 4-cm irregular mass (*A*). Core needle biopsy confirmed invasive ductal carcinoma. An MRI was performed revealing a mass in the posterior breast (*B*) corresponding to the mass seen on sonography. There was loss of the fat plane posteriorly with enhancement of the muscle, indicative of chest wall invasion. The patient underwent neoadjuvant chemotherapy before surgery.

disease in patients requiring mastectomy but desiring breast conservation. Before surgery, systemic therapy may be given in an attempt to shrink the tumor.[45,46] Complete pathologic response is associated with favorable prognosis. Patients who fail to respond must be identified early, so that alterations may be made in the treatment plan.

However, monitoring response to the chemotherapy may be difficult. There are limitations in following patients on clinical breast examination and on mammography. Breast density may limit the mammographic evaluation, and fibrotic

changes may limit the clinical breast examination. Breast ultrasound may be a feasible option for a solitary lesion but may be of limited use in evaluating very large cancers or multifocal or multicentric cancers. It may also be difficult to differentiate necrotic tumor from viable tumor on sonography (**Fig. 10**). Breast MRI is ideal in following patients because the limitations with density and fibrosis do not affect the evaluation. Because MRI imaging depends on vascularity, nonviable necrotic tissue will not enhance. In addition, a global assessment of the breast may be made (**Fig. 11**). MRI can assess for volume change and evaluate the

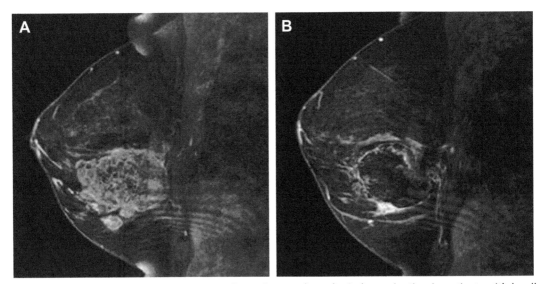

Fig. 10. MRI may better estimate response to chemotherapy than physical examination in patients with locally advanced breast cancer. MRI shows a large microlobulated mass in the inferior breast (*A*). After 4 cycles of chemotherapy, the overall size had not changed significantly, but the central portion of the mass did not enhance in keeping with necrosis (*B*).

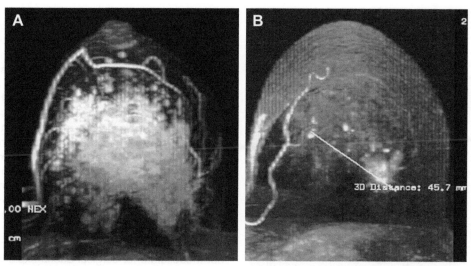

Fig. 11. A patient with locally advanced breast cancer. MRI was obtained shortly after presentation (A). After neoadjuvant chemotherapy, there was marked decrease in tumor size (B).

pattern of response. Studies have shown that decreased enhancement on MRI correlates with a positive response to chemotherapy and with residual disease at pathology, whereas minimal or no change or enlargement of the cancer on MRI correlates with lack of response.[47–50] Recent reports suggest that the pattern of response on MRI may hold important predictive information, but further studies need to be done.

Although MRI can assess for macroscopic disease, it cannot evaluate for microscopic foci. Although the patient may have complete imaging response on MRI, at surgery extensive microscopic disease or rests of tumor cells below the threshold of MRI may be present. There are reports that treatment with taxane-related chemotherapeutic agents can lead to underestimation of residual cancer on MRI, possibly because of decreased vascularity. The author's team at the University of Pennsylvania advocates placement of a clip before neoadjuvant therapy to facilitate localizing the original tumor site for excisional biopsy if there is complete imaging response.

Studies have also shown that evaluation of the choline peak may serve as a marker for therapy response.[51–53] Choline, an essential component of the cell membrane, can be measured using MR spectroscopy. Studies have shown that a decrease in the choline peak may serve as an early marker of tumor response. The choline peak may decrease soon after administration of chemotherapy, before any gross tumor morphologic changes are evident on MRI.[52] Meisamy and colleagues[52] measured levels of choline-containing compounds using spectroscopy on a 4T

magnet before and after administration of chemotherapy in 14 patients. The first postchemotherapy study was obtained within 24 hours of the dose. Another follow-up MRI was obtained after the fourth dose. Meisamy and colleagues found that the change in choline levels from baseline compared with the first posttreatment study differed significantly between the responders and the nonresponders. Baek and colleagues[53] at the University of California at Irvine did not detect significant differences in choline concentrations between complete responders and noncomplete responders after the first dose of chemotherapy. However, the authors have found choline concentration levels midway through therapy to be a better predictor of response. After analyzing many variables, the authors found the tumor size at mid therapy to be overall the best predictor of response.

Unknown Primary

Presentation of clinically and mammographically occult breast cancer with a positive axillary lymph node is an uncommon event, accounting for less than 1% of diagnosed breast cancers (Fig. 12). Traditionally, the treatment of choice has been mastectomy and axillary node dissection. Even after mastectomy, the primary cancer was only found one third of the time, with no survival difference between women who did and did not have mastectomy.

Reports of MRI-detected primaries were published in the late 1990s with additional articles supporting the findings of the original articles. The

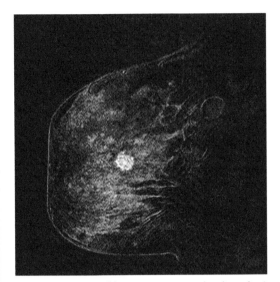

Fig. 12. A 44-year-old woman presented to her physician with left axillary node enlargement. Fine-needle aspiration revealed adenocarcinoma. Mammography and physical exam were negative. The patient subsequently had an MRI examination that revealed an enhancing mass in the left breast. Biopsy confirmed a breast primary.

reported MRI sensitivity varies from 25% to 100%.[54–57] The largest series was by Buchanan[57] and colleagues in 2005, and it reported a 59% detection rate in 162 patients. Once the primary is detected on MRI, the area may be biopsied under MR guidance or possibly under ultrasound guidance if it is visible on second-look ultrasound, and the patient may be a candidate for breast conservation therapy if there is localized disease. At the University of Pennsylvania, if the MRI fails to demonstrate the primary cancer, the patient is offered the option of mastectomy with or without reconstruction or whole breast radiation.

Evaluation of Nipple Discharge

Unilateral spontaneous nipple discharge that is bloody, clear, or serosanguinous may be an early clinical manifestation of breast cancer. Approximately 5% to 20% of patients presenting with such symptoms will have breast cancer, although the most common cause will be papillomas. Conventional imaging methods, such as mammography and ultrasound, are limited in the evaluation of nipple discharge. Cytologic evaluation of the discharge fluid is also limited. Mammography, however, needs to be performed to assess for any unsuspected masses or calcifications. In addition to mammography, MRI may also have a role in evaluating patients with

clinically significant nipple discharge (**Fig. 13**).[58–61] Various studies have reported MRI may be able demonstrate cancer that is occult on clinical breast exam and on conventional imaging.[58–60] In a retrospective study, Morrogh and colleagues[58] retrospectively evaluated the PPV of MRI and of galactography in patients presenting with clinically significant nipple discharge and negative clinical breast examination, mammography, and sonography. The PPV of galactography and MRI were 19% and 56%, respectively. The negative predictive value (NPV) of galactography and MRI were 63% and 87%, respectively. Although MRI had a higher PPV than galactography in detection of breast cancer, the authors concluded that a negative MRI did not exclude malignancy, given its NPV of 87%. It was also not a substitute for surgical ductal exploration in the appropriate clinical setting.

Abnormal Mammogram

MRI may be used as a problem-solving tool once conventional imaging methods have been exhausted with equivocal results. However, MRI must not be used as a substitute for a suboptimal conventional workup. One situation in which an MRI may be helpful is in the case of focal asymmetry, or a finding seen with only one view on a mammogram, with no sonographic correlate. If the corresponding lesion enhances, MRI may help to localize the lesion for biopsy. In such situations, it is essential that MRI-mammographic correlation be made to ensure that the MRI lesion

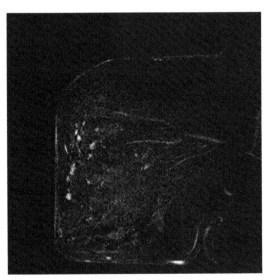

Fig. 13. Patient presenting with a history of bloody nipple discharge. Mammography was negative. MRI shows multiple small enhancing masses in the subareolar region. Biopsy revealed papillomas.

corresponds to the mammographic lesion. A targeted second-look ultrasound may also be performed to assess if the lesion is sonographically visible, and if the lesion is visible, ultrasound-guided biopsy is a feasible option. It is the practice at the University of Pennsylvania when a MRI is recommended for additional evaluation to give management recommendations based on the conventional imaging findings in the mammogram/ultrasound report. If there is no MRI correlate for the mammographic finding, there is then a clear plan of action in the mammogram report whether it is routine follow-up, short-term follow-up, or biopsy. This prevents the MRI reader from re-interpreting the mammogram and/or the ultrasound studies and second guessing the initial interpreting radiologist. This also gives the ordering clinician clear guidelines for the management of the patient should the MRI be negative.

Although the sensitivity of MRI for invasive cancer is high, a suspicious finding on conventional imaging should not preclude biopsy based on a negative MRI.

High-risk Screening

Although mammography has been established as the primary screening tool for breast cancer, the sensitivity of mammography is limited, particularly in women with dense breast tissue. Although the lifetime breast cancer risk for a woman is 1 out of 8, for a mutation carrier the lifetime risk can be as high as 80%.[62,63] In addition to significantly higher lifetime risk, these women tend to develop more aggressive cancers at an earlier age (**Fig. 14**). Many studies have reported mammographically occult breast cancer detected on MRI in high-risk populations.[3,9–16,64]

Kriege and colleagues[3] screened 1909 women with greater than 15% lifetime risk for breast cancer, comparing clinical breast examination every 6 months with annual mammography and MRI. A total of 358 women were known BRCA carriers. The sensitivity and specificity of each of the examinations for invasive cancer were as follows, respectively: clinical breast examination, 17.9%, 98.1%; mammography, 33.3%, 95.0%; and MRI, 79.5%, 89.8%. Although MRI had higher sensitivity in detecting invasive cancer, it was at the cost of slightly decreased specificity.

In the United Kingdom, Leach and colleagues[9] screened 649 women who had a strong family history of breast cancer or were known BRCA or TP53 mutation carriers. The women were screened with mammography and MRI. Thirty-five cancers were diagnosed in 649 women, 19 were seen only on MRI, 6 only on mammography,

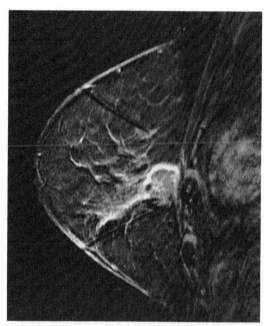

Fig. 14. A 48-year-old *BRCA1*-positive patient who underwent annual MRI screening. The patient's annual MRI examination demonstrated an enhancing mass in the posterior breast with linear enhancement extending anteriorly. Biopsy revealed a high-grade invasive ductal carcinoma. The patient underwent neoadjuvant chemotherapy before mastectomy.

8 on both mammography and MRI, and 2 were interval cases. The sensitivity and specificity for MRI were 77% and 81%, respectively, and for mammography, 40% and 93%, respectively. The combined sensitivity of MRI and mammography was 94%. Thirteen of the 35 cancers were diagnosed in *BRCA1* carriers, and it is in this group that MRI sensitivity was the greatest, 92% for MRI versus 23% for mammography.

Kuhl and colleagues[64] prospectively screened 529 asymptomatic high-risk women detecting 43 cancers, 34 invasive cancers and 9 DCIS. There was 1 interval cancer. The sensitivity and specificity were 91% and 97.2%, respectively, for MRI and 33% and 96.8%, respectively, for mammography. In the known mutation carriers, the sensitivity of MRI and mammography were, respectively, 100% and 25%. MRI detected 14 invasive cancers and 5 intraductal cancers.

Canadian results also confirm the higher sensitivity of MRI compared with mammography. Warner and colleagues[11] screened 236 women, detecting 22 cancers (16 invasive and 6 DCIS). The sensitivity and specificity were, respectively, 77% and 95.4% for MRI and 33% and 99.8% for mammography.

Screening trials have confirmed that MRI has higher sensitivity than mammography in detecting occult cancers. Based on prior studies, the sensitivity of MRI ranges from 71% to 100% compared with 16% to 40% for mammography,[8] with some studies indicating that MRI can even detect mammographically occult DCIS. The higher sensitivity of MRI is obtained at the cost of a higher biopsy rate or a lower specificity. The specificity of MRI is consistently lower than the specificity of mammography. In addition, there is lack of data demonstrating that MRI screening will ultimately result in a lower recurrence rate or improved survival for these patients. A large randomized study with mortality as the endpoint would be needed to answer such a question, but such a study would be extremely expensive and difficult to perform and therefore will probably never be done.

Based on available data, the American Cancer Society's guidelines for screening includes annual MRI screening for women who have greater than 20% to 25% lifetime risk for breast cancer.[8] Based on evidence from screening trials and observational studies, screening is recommended for women with known BRCA mutations, women who are first-degree but untested relatives of known carriers, and women with a greater than 20% to 25% lifetime risk based on risk assessment models that are primarily dependent on family history. Based on expert consensus opinion, annual MRI is recommended for patients with Cowden syndrome, Bannayan-Riley-Ruvalcaba syndrome, and Li-Fraumeni syndrome and their first-degree relatives and for women who received radiation therapy to the chest between ages 10 and 30 years. It is thought that there is inconclusive evidence regarding MRI screening of women with a personal history of breast cancer, lobular carcinoma in situ, atypical lobular hyperplasia, atypical ductal carcinoma, dense breast tissue, and lifetime risk levels of 15% to 20%. Based on expert opinion, MRI is not recommended for women with less than 15% lifetime risk of breast cancer.

Controversies

Criticisms about MRI imaging include its potential for a high false-positive rate, leading to unnecessary biopsies, and the clinical relevance of MRI-detected cancers. There are many factors that contribute to the false-positive rate. One is the interobserver variability in the radiologists interpreting the MRI studies,[65,66] which is also observed in mammogram interpretations.[67] It is to be hoped that as experience with breast MRI increases, the false-positive rate will decrease. Studies have shown

and it has been our experience at the University of Pennsylvania that in the screening setting, the recall rate decreases with subsequent rounds of screening.[10,68] Comparison studies will decrease the recall rate, as also seen with mammography. The latest edition of the American College of Radiology Breast Imaging Reporting and Data System includes a lexicon for breast MRI.[69] Developments are also underway to standardize the protocol for breast MRI image acquisition. As the lexicon and the imaging guidelines become standardized, variations in technique and interpretation will decrease.

Another common criticism of MRI is the clinical relevance of the cancer that is detected. Prior studies reporting pathologic evaluation of mastectomy specimens have shown additional tumor foci separate from the known primary tumor in 38% to 54% of patients.[38,70] The presence of unsuspected residual tumor foci of pathologic evaluation was, in the past, used as an argument against breast conservation therapy. However, Smitt and colleagues[71] reported local recurrence after breast conservation therapy at 10 years to be less than 10% in patients with negative surgical margins. It has been argued that whole breast radiation "controlled" residual disease that may be present. As localized treatment, such as partial breast radiation, gains popularity, it remains to be seen if MRI will play a greater role in treatment planning.

There is evidence from many studies that MRI detects clinically and mammographically occult breast cancer. However, there are no prospective randomized studies showing improved long-term or disease-free survival or reduced recurrence rates in women who undergo breast MRI. And it is doubtful if such a study could be done. To answer these questions, the study would need to enroll a large number of patients (to achieve statistical significance) with long follow-up, which would make such a study very expensive to perform.

SUMMARY

In the past 2 decades, contrast-enhanced breast MRI has become an integral component of breast imaging. Over the years, improvements in MRI technology and biopsy capability have resulted in diagnosing mammographically and clinically occult breast cancer. The clinical indications for breast MRI will continue to evolve and expand in the future.

REFERENCES

1. Jemal A, Siegel R, Ward E, et al. Cancer statistics, 2009. CA Cancer J Clin 2009;59:225.

2. Kerlikowske K, Carney PA, Geller B, et al. Performance of screening mammography among women with and without a first-degree relative with breast cancer. Ann Intern Med 2000;133:855.

3. Kriege M, Brekelmans CT, Boetes C, et al. Efficacy of MRI and mammography for breast-cancer screening in women with a familial or genetic predisposition. N Engl J Med 2004;351:427.

4. Mandelson MT, Oestreicher N, Porter PL, et al. Breast density as a predictor of mammographic detection: comparison of interval- and screen-detected cancers. J Natl Cancer Inst 2000;92:1081.

5. Kuhl CK. The "coming of age" of nonmammographic screening for breast cancer. JAMA 2008;299:2203.

6. Kaiser WA, Zeitler E. MR imaging of the breast: fast imaging sequences with and without Gd-DTPA. Preliminary observations. Radiology 1989;170:681.

7. Heywang SH, Wolf A, Pruss E, et al. MR imaging of the breast with Gd-DTPA: use and limitations. Radiology 1989;171:95.

8. Saslow D, Boetes C, Burke W, et al. American Cancer Society guidelines for breast screening with MRI as an adjunct to mammography. CA Cancer J Clin 2007;57:75.

9. Leach MO, Boggis CR, Dixon AK, et al. Screening with magnetic resonance imaging and mammography of a UK population at high familial risk of breast cancer: a prospective multicentre cohort study (MARIBS). Lancet 2005;365:1769.

10. Kuhl CK, Schmutzler RK, Leutner CC, et al. Breast MR imaging screening in 192 women proved or suspected to be carriers of a breast cancer susceptibility gene: preliminary results. Radiology 2000;215:267.

11. Warner E, Plewes DB, Hill KA, et al. Surveillance of BRCA1 and BRCA2 mutation carriers with magnetic resonance imaging, ultrasound, mammography, and clinical breast examination. JAMA 2004;292:1317.

12. Podo F, Sardanelli F, Canese R, et al. The Italian multicentre project on evaluation of MRI and other imaging modalities in early detection of breast cancer in subjects at high genetic risk. J Exp Clin Cancer Res 2002;21:115.

13. Tilanus-Linthorst MM, Obdeijn IM, Bartels KC, et al. First experiences in screening women at high risk for breast cancer with MR imaging. Breast Cancer Res Treat 2000;63:53.

14. Morris EA, Liberman L, Ballon DJ, et al. MRI of occult breast carcinoma in a high-risk population. AJR Am J Roentgenol 2003;181:619.

15. Lehman CD, Blume JD, Weatherall P, et al. Screening women at high risk for breast cancer with mammography and magnetic resonance imaging. Cancer 2005;103:1898.

16. Lehman CD, Isaacs C, Schnall MD, et al. Cancer yield of mammography, MR, and US in high-risk women: prospective multi-institution breast cancer screening study. Radiology 2007;244:381.

17. Kuhl CK, Schrading S, Bieling HB, et al. MRI for diagnosis of pure ductal carcinoma in situ: a prospective observational study. Lancet 2007; 370:485.

18. Orel SG, Schnall MD. MR imaging of the breast for the detection, diagnosis, and staging of breast cancer. Radiology 2001;220:13.

19. Schnall MD, Blume J, Bluemke DA, et al. MRI detection of distinct incidental cancer in women with primary breast cancer studied in IBMC 6883. J Surg Oncol 2005;92:32.

20. Deurloo EE, Peterse JL, Rutgers EJ, et al. Additional breast lesions in patients eligible for breast-conserving therapy by MRI: impact on preoperative management and potential benefit of computerised analysis. Eur J Cancer 2005;41:1393.

21. Schelfout K, Van Goethem M, Kersschot E, et al. Contrast-enhanced MR imaging of breast lesions and effect on treatment. Eur J Surg Oncol 2004;30:501.

22. Berg WA, Gutierrez L, NessAiver MS, et al. Diagnostic accuracy of mammography, clinical examination, US, and MR imaging in preoperative assessment of breast cancer. Radiology 2004;233:830.

23. Hata T, Takahashi H, Watanabe K, et al. Magnetic resonance imaging for preoperative evaluation of breast cancer: a comparative study with mammography and ultrasonography. J Am Coll Surg 2004; 198:190.

24. Sardanelli F, Giuseppetti GM, Panizza P, et al. Sensitivity of MRI versus mammography for detecting foci of multifocal, multicentric breast cancer in Fatty and dense breasts using the whole-breast pathologic examination as a gold standard. AJR Am J Roentgenol 2004;183:1149.

25. Menell JH, Morris EA, Dershaw DD, et al. Determination of the presence and extent of pure ductal carcinoma in situ by mammography and magnetic resonance imaging. Breast J 2005;11:382.

26. Fisher B, Anderson S, Bryant J, et al. Twenty-year follow-up of a randomized trial comparing total mastectomy, lumpectomy, and lumpectomy plus irradiation for the treatment of invasive breast cancer. N Engl J Med 2002;347:1233.

27. Veronesi U, Cascinelli N, Mariani L, et al. Twenty-year follow-up of a randomized study comparing breast-conserving surgery with radical mastectomy for early breast cancer. N Engl J Med 2002;347: 1227.

28. Clarke M, Collins R, Darby S, et al. Effects of radiotherapy and of differences in the extent of surgery for early breast cancer on local recurrence and 15-year survival: an overview of the randomised trials. Lancet 2005;366:2087.

29. Schwartz GF, Veronesi U, Clough KB, et al. Proceedings of the consensus conference on breast conservation, April 28 to May 1, 2005, Milan, Italy. Cancer 2006;107:242.

30. Wapnir IL, Anderson SJ, Mamounas EP, et al. Prognosis after ipsilateral breast tumor recurrence and locoregional recurrences in five National Surgical Adjuvant Breast and Bowel Project node-positive adjuvant breast cancer trials. J Clin Oncol 2006; 24:2028.

31. Orel SG, Schnall MD, Powell CM, et al. Staging of suspected breast cancer: effect of MR imaging and MR-guided biopsy. Radiology 1995;196:115.

32. Fischer U, Kopka L, Grabbe E. Breast carcinoma: effect of preoperative contrast-enhanced MR imaging on the therapeutic approach. Radiology 1999;213:881.

33. Boetes C, Mus RD, Holland R, et al. Breast tumors: comparative accuracy of MR imaging relative to mammography and US for demonstrating extent. Radiology 1995;197:743.

34. Mumtaz H, Hall-Craggs MA, Davidson T, et al. Staging of symptomatic primary breast cancer with MR imaging. AJR Am J Roentgenol 1997;169:417.

35. Kramer S, Schulz-Wendtland R, Hagedorn K, et al. Magnetic resonance imaging and its role in the diagnosis of multicentric breast cancer. Anticancer Res 1998;18:2163.

36. Faverly DR, Hendriks JH, Holland R. Breast carcinomas of limited extent: frequency, radiologic-pathologic characteristics, and surgical margin requirements. Cancer 2001;91:647.

37. Holland R, Veling SH, Mravunac M, et al. Histologic multifocality of Tis, T1-2 breast carcinomas. Implications for clinical trials of breast-conserving surgery. Cancer 1985;56:979.

38. Rosen PP, Fracchia AA, Urban JA, et al. "Residual" mammary carcinoma following simulated partial mastectomy. Cancer 1975;35:739.

39. Fisher B, Anderson S, Redmond CK, et al. Reanalysis and results after 12 years of follow-up in a randomized clinical trial comparing total mastectomy with lumpectomy with or without irradiation in the treatment of breast cancer. N Engl J Med 1995;333:1456.

40. Veronesi U, Luini A, Galimberti V, et al. Conservation approaches for the management of stage I/II carcinoma of the breast: Milan Cancer Institute trials. World J Surg 1994;18:70.

41. Veronesi U, Luini A, Del Vecchio M, et al. Radiotherapy after breast-preserving surgery in women with localized cancer of the breast. N Engl J Med 1993;328:1587.

42. Bedrosian I, Mick R, Orel SG, et al. Changes in the surgical management of patients with breast carcinoma based on preoperative magnetic resonance imaging. Cancer 2003;98:468.

43. Morris EA, Schwartz LH, Drotman MB, et al. Evaluation of pectoralis major muscle in patients with posterior breast tumors on breast MR images: early experience. Radiology 2000;214:67.

44. Kazama T, Nakamura S, Doi O, et al. Prospective evaluation of pectoralis muscle invasion of breast cancer by MR imaging. Breast Cancer 2005;12:312.

45. Fisher B, Brown A, Mamounas E, et al. Effect of preoperative chemotherapy on local-regional disease in women with operable breast cancer: findings from National Surgical Adjuvant Breast and Bowel Project B-18. J Clin Oncol 1997;15:2483.

46. Fisher B, Bryant J, Wolmark N, et al. Effect of preoperative chemotherapy on the outcome of women with operable breast cancer. J Clin Oncol 1998;16:2672.

47. Chang YC, Huang CS, Liu YJ, et al. Angiogenic response of locally advanced breast cancer to neoadjuvant chemotherapy evaluated with parametric histogram from dynamic contrast-enhanced MRI. Phys Med Biol 2004;49:3593.

48. Martincich L, Montemurro F, De Rosa G, et al. Monitoring response to primary chemotherapy in breast cancer using dynamic contrast-enhanced magnetic resonance imaging. Breast Cancer Res Treat 2004; 83:67.

49. Padhani AR, Hayes C, Assersohn L, et al. Prediction of clinicopathologic response of breast cancer to primary chemotherapy at contrast-enhanced MR imaging: initial clinical results. Radiology 2006;239: 361.

50. Pickles MD, Lowry M, Manton DJ, et al. Role of dynamic contrast enhanced MRI in monitoring early response of locally advanced breast cancer to neoadjuvant chemotherapy. Breast Cancer Res Treat 2005;91:1.

51. Jagannathan NR, Kumar M, Seenu V, et al. Evaluation of total choline from in-vivo volume localized proton MR spectroscopy and its response to neoadjuvant chemotherapy in locally advanced breast cancer. Br J Cancer 2001;84:1016.

52. Meisamy S, Bolan PJ, Baker EH, et al. Neoadjuvant chemotherapy of locally advanced breast cancer: predicting response with in vivo (1)H MR spectroscopy–a pilot study at 4 T. Radiology 2004;233:424.

53. Baek HM, Chen JH, Nie K, et al. Predicting pathologic response to neoadjuvant chemotherapy in breast cancer by using MR imaging and quantitative 1H MR spectroscopy. Radiology 2009;251:653.

54. Orel SG, Weinstein SP, Schnall MD, et al. Breast MR imaging in patients with axillary node metastases and unknown primary malignancy. Radiology 1999; 212:543–9.

55. Morris EA, Schwartz LH, Dershaw DD, et al. MR imaging of the breast in patients with occult primary breast carcinoma. Radiology 1997;205:437.

56. Tilanus-Linthorst MM, Obdeijn AI, Bontenbal M, et al. MRI in patients with axillary metastases of occult breast carcinoma. Breast Cancer Res Treat 1997;44:179–82.

57. Buchanan CL, Morris EA, Dorn PL, et al. Utility of breast magnetic resonance imaging in patients

with occult primary breast cancer. Ann Surg Oncol 2005;12:1045.

58. Morrogh M, Morris EA, Liberman L, et al. The predictive value of ductography and magnetic resonance imaging in the management of nipple discharge. Ann Surg Oncol 2007;14:3369.

59. Orel SG, Dougherty CS, Reynolds C, et al. MR imaging in patients with nipple discharge: initial experience. Radiology 2000;216:248.

60. Nakahara H, Namba K, Watanabe R, et al. A comparison of MR imaging, galactography and ultrasonography in patients with nipple discharge. Breast Cancer 2003;10:320.

61. Yoshimoto M, Kasumi F, Iwase T, et al. Magnetic resonance galactography for a patient with nipple discharge. Breast Cancer Res Treat 1997;42:87.

62. Ford D, Easton DF, Bishop DT, et al. Risks of cancer in BRCA1-mutation carriers. Breast Cancer Linkage Consortium. Lancet 1994;343:692.

63. Antoniou A, Pharoah PD, Narod S, et al. Average risks of breast and ovarian cancer associated with BRCA1 or BRCA2 mutations detected in case Series unselected for family history: a combined analysis of 22 studies. Am J Hum Genet 2003;72:1117.

64. Kuhl CK, Schrading S, Leutner CC, et al. Mammography, breast ultrasound, and magnetic resonance imaging for surveillance of women at high familial risk for breast cancer. J Clin Oncol 2005;23:8469.

65. Warren RM, Pointon L, Thompson D, et al. Reading protocol for dynamic contrast-enhanced MR images of the breast: sensitivity and specificity analysis. Radiology 2005;236:779.

66. Ikeda DM, Hylton NM, Kinkel K, et al. Development, standardization, and testing of a lexicon for reporting contrast-enhanced breast magnetic resonance imaging studies. J Magn Reson Imaging 2001;13:889.

67. Berg WA, Campassi C, Langenberg P, et al. Breast Imaging Reporting and Data System: inter- and intraobserver variability in feature analysis and final assessment. AJR Am J Roentgenol 2000;174:1769.

68. Warner E, Causer PA. MRI surveillance for hereditary breast-cancer risk. Lancet 2005;365:1747.

69. American College of Radiology. ACR Breast Imaging Reporting and Data System, Breast Imaging Atlas. Reston (VA): American College of Radiology; 2003.

70. Qualheim RE, Gall EA. Breast carcinoma with multiple sites of origin. Cancer 1957;10:460.

71. Smitt MC, Nowels KW, Zdeblick MJ, et al. The importance of the lumpectomy surgical margin status in long-term results of breast conservation. Cancer 1995;76:259.

FDG-PET Dynamic Contrast-Enhanced CT in the Management of Breast Cancer

Chandan J. Das, MD[a], Abeer Al-Mullah, MD[b],
Rakesh Kumar, MD[c],*

KEYWORDS
- Breast cancer • FDG • PET • CT

Breast cancer is the most common cancer and second only to lung and bronchial cancer as a cause of cancer death in women. In 2009, an estimated 192,370 new cases of female breast cancer will be diagnosed and 40,170 patients will die of breast cancer in the United States.[1] Early diagnosis and reliable imaging assessment of response to treatment are essential in the clinical management of breast cancer.

Management of breast cancer is a multidisciplinary approach that includes surgery, chemotherapy, hormonal modulation, and radiation therapy. Neoadjuvant chemotherapy also provides an exciting options for breast conservation.[2] The current system of providing a choice between mastectomy and breast conservation surgery is economically viable.[3]

Breast conservation therapy should be considered the preferred surgical option for most women who have early operable breast cancer. Adjuvant systemic chemotherapy or hormonal therapy can substantially reduce the risk for recurrence and death. Neoadjuvant chemotherapy or primary systemic therapy in operable breast cancer slightly increases the incidence of breast conservation.[4] Breast conservation therapy with segmental mastectomy and postoperative radiation therapy with or without axillary lymph node dissection provides excellent local control and disease-free survival in elderly women who have breast carcinoma.[5]

The recognition of HER2 as a prognostic factor and target for treatment further widens the range of therapeutic options in breast cancer.[6] Developments in the field of surgery, breast irradiation, newer chemotherapeutic drugs, and hormonal and biologic agents further expand the possibilities for breast conservation. This paradigm shift in treatment options demands efficient early diagnostic and follow-up imaging techniques.

CURRENT IMAGING OPTIONS

Although numerous advances and improvements have been made in the field of breast imaging in the past decade, mammography is still the most widely used technique for the early detection and diagnosis of breast cancer because of its diagnostic value, patient compliance, and low costs.[7] Mammography also has an appropriate role in breast cancer follow-up in the setting of adjuvant chemotherapy. Ultrasonography is predominantly used to evaluate a dense breast, characterize an undetermined lesion on mammography, evaluate axillary lymph nodes, and guide needle aspiration for pathologic diagnosis. Advances in imaging technologies have resulted in exciting techniques in breast imaging, including digital mammography,

Portions of this article were previously published in: Kumar R, Das CJ. Hybrid PET-dynamic CECT in the management of breast cancer. Eur J Nucl Med Mol Imaging 2009;36(3):413–6.

[a] Department of Radiology, All India Institute of Medical Sciences, New Delhi, India
[b] Department of Medical Imaging, King Fahd Specialist Hospital, Dammam, Kingdom of Saudi Arabia
[c] Department of Nuclear Medicine, All India Institute of Medical Sciences, New Delhi, India
* Corresponding author.
E-mail address: rkphulia@yahoo.com (R. Kumar).

PET Clin 4 (2009) 255–263
doi:10.1016/j.cpet.2009.09.005

MRI coupled with diffusion-weighted imaging (DWI), computer-aided diagnosis, single-photon emission planar CT imaging (SPECT), PET, and hybrid PET-CT imaging.

Computer-aided detection technology with full-field digital mammography has been effective in helping radiologists with early detection of breast cancer.[8] MRI may compete with fluorodeoxyglucose (FDG)-PET as far as ionizing radiation is considered. Dynamic contrast-enhanced MRI has been established as a valuable tool for detecting breast cancer. Dynamic enhanced magnetic resonance mammography has a high sensitivity of 86% to 96%, a specificity of 64% to 91%, an accuracy of 79% to 93%, a positive predictive value of 77% to 92%, and a negative predictive value of 75% to 94% for detecting breast cancer, but also a high false-positive diagnosis rate.[9]

Growing evidence suggests the plausible role of DWI in the management of breast cancer. DWI has a high sensitivity for detecting breast tumors, especially those that are malignant. DWI is highly sensitive in detecting malignant breast lesions even with qualitative assessment alone, whereas apparent coefficient diffusion measurement offers quantitative assessment and increases the specificity to more than 90%.[10] Early study using a rabbit metastatic breast cancer model showed that MRI is superior to 18F-deoxyglucose (FDG)-PET/CT in monitoring tumor metastasis.[11]

The most commonly explored nuclear medicine techniques are FDG-PET scan with FDG-PET and SPECT. Other functional radionuclide-based diagnostic tools include scintimammography with sestamibi, peptide scintigraphy, and immunoscintigraphy. Conventional imaging modalities, such as screen-film mammography, digital mammography, ultrasonography, and MRI, provide only morphologic details and not information on the metabolic status of a lesion, which is important in differentiating benign lesions from malignant, and therefore conventional imaging modalities lack specificity.

During the past decade, FDG-PET has been widely shown to be highly useful for the diagnosing palpable masses, staging, long-term follow-up, and showing tumor response to chemotherapy at an early phase or after completion of treatment in patients who have breast cancer. However, like other nuclear medicine techniques, it also has poor anatomic resolution.

Visual correlation of FDG-PET with morphologic procedures, such as CT, has been shown to improve the accuracy of FDG-PET alone. With advances in technology, the spatial resolution has been enhanced by introduction of the hybrid FDG-PET/CT scanner, in which the FDG-PET part of the scanner is equipped with a high-resolution state-of-the-art multidetector CT (MDCT) system for simultaneous acquisition of the FDG-PET and CT data. CT contrast can be injected to get the standard contrast-enhanced image. Introduction of this hybrid FDG-PET/CT scanner has expanded the possibilities for oncologic imaging, and has been projected to be a "one-stop shop" for not only for diagnosing the primary lesion but also determining metastasis to various organs.

Individually performed FDG-PET scans and contrast-enhanced CT (CECT) have important roles imaging breast cancer. Because of the increased experience with FDG-PET/CT over the past several years, this article explores the role of FDG-PET/CECT performed in this setting using a hybrid FDG-PET/CT scanner. This article attempts to tease out the role of FDG-PET/CECT in the management of breast cancer, and discusses the applicability of this technique.

ROLE OF FDG-PET IN BREAST CANCER

Published literature suggests that FDG-PET has become an efficient tumor diagnostic tool because of its outstanding sensitivity and specificity. It is a useful and cost-beneficial diagnostic modality when used within its limitations. FDG-PET is complementary to conventional staging procedures and can provide additional information when results of conventional imaging are indeterminate or of limited usefulness. For breast cancer, FDG-PET often shows locoregional or unsuspected distant disease and is particularly helpful for evaluating chemotherapy response in patients who have locally advanced breast carcinoma and those who have metastatic disease.[12]

STAGING

Whole body FDG-PET can provide functional information that is not provided by anatomic imaging modalities such as CT or mammography, and can help narrow the differential diagnosis of breast masses, stage the cancer, and monitor patients posttreatment.[9,13] FDG-PET has an important role in predicting tumor response in patients who have locally advanced breast cancer undergoing neoadjuvant chemotherapy, and differentiating scar tissue from cancer recurrence.[9,14] FDG uptake may represent a surrogate marker of tumor biology in patients who have proven primary breast cancer with varying disease burden at diagnosis.[15]

FDG-PET is not a very useful modality for screening and early diagnosis of breast carcinoma. The sensitivity of FDG-PET is 92% for lesions larger than 20 mm, but is only 53% for primary lesions smaller than 5 mm.[16] This poor detection of small lesions is a result of partial volume effects and low FDG uptake in the tumor compared with the background breast tissue.[16]

The status of axillary lymph nodes (ALNs) is the most important prognostic factor in breast cancer.[17] FDG-PET has shown efficacy in detecting ALN metastases. Even in some clinical trials its accuracy proved nearly comparable to that of lymphoscintigraphy with sentinel node biopsy, whereas other studies showed that FDG-PET scanning does not have adequate spatial resolution to detect both micro- and small macrometastatic disease in ALNs. FDG-PET can improve staging and alter therapeutic options primarily by showing local or distant nodal involvement not seen on other imaging studies. FDG-PET is superior to conventional imaging procedures for detecting distant metastases, and CT is complementary to FDG-PET.[18] On a lesion basis, FDG-PET detects significantly more lymph nodes but fewer bone metastases than conventional imaging. The high predictive value of FDG-PET can change the tumor stage and may lead to modification of therapeutic strategy.[19]

ADVANTAGES AND PITFALLS

FDG-PET has been evaluated in breast cancer for the characterization of primary tumors, lymph node staging, and follow-up of patients after surgery, chemotherapy, or radiotherapy. In contrast to the low sensitivity and moderate specificity of FDG-PET in the initial detection and characterization of breast cancer, and its low lesion-based sensitivity for lymph node staging, the results from FDG-PET use in restaging of patients who have breast cancer are promising.

A major advantage of FDG-PET imaging compared with conventional imaging is that it screens the entire patient for local recurrence, lymph node metastases, and distant metastases during a single whole-body examination, with a reported average sensitivity and specificity of 96% and 77%, respectively.[20] Apart from cost, other limitations of FDG-PET in the follow-up of patients who have breast cancer include its relatively low detection rate of bone metastases, especially the blastic subtype. The rather low specificity of FDG-PET can be increased by using FDG-PET/CT imaging.

ROLE OF FDG-PET/CT

Imaging techniques such as CT and MRI provide excellent anatomic details but not information on metabolic activity of the tumors. With the advent of a hybrid FDG-PET/CT scanner, information on morphology and functional activity of the tumors can be obtained simultaneously. The merging of the two techniques has replaced the need for separate FDG-PET and CT examinations. The hybrid FDG-PET/CT system has advantages over separate FDG-PET and CT examinations for detecting distant metastases and recurrences, and for monitoring treatment response. The hybrid FDG-PET/CT has shown that the two techniques are adding their potentialities.[21] Combined FDG-PET/CT seemed to be more accurate in assessing the TNM and showed a moderate impact on therapy compared with FDG-PET and CT.[22]

FDG-PET/CT has changed the scenario of breast cancer management during the past few years by providing accurate evaluation of morphology through its CT component and depicting abnormal metabolic activity through its PET component. However, FDG-PET/CT has limited diagnostic value for detecting small primary breast tumors and well-differentiated breast cancer, but this can be improved using dual time point scan.[23] FDG-PET/CT is not a reliable modality for assessing axillary lymph node, although it is invaluable tool for assessing unsuspected extra-axillary lymph nodes and distant metastases.[17,24,25] The reported sensitivity and specificity of FDG-PET/CT in detecting axillary lymph nodes metastases are 70% and 100%, respectively.[25]

FDG-PET/CT may extend the indication for sentinel lymph node biopsy (SLNB) and enhances the identification rates of sentinel nodes, thus increasing the accuracy of SLNB.[26–28] However, when the axillary staging cannot be performed with ultrasonography alone, FDG-PET/CT may be used for final staging.[29] Overall sensitivity and specificity of FDG-PET/CT for detecting distant metastases are 100% and 98%, respectively.[25,30]

FDG-PET/CT provides additional information on locoregional and distant metastasis in patients who have inflammatory breast cancer.[31] FDG-PET/CT only marginally improves the restaging accuracy over FDG-PET alone in patients who have breast cancer.[32] FDG-PET/CT allows early prediction of the response to chemotherapy in patient who have locally advanced breast cancer and can differentiate responders from non-responders with high accuracy after two cycles of neoadjuvant chemotherapy in patients who have locally advanced breast cancer.[33]

FDG-PET/CT imaging is closely related to cell apoptosis status of breast cancer after neoadjuvant chemotherapy, and may be applied to predict treatment response.[34] The main advantage of FDG-PET/CT over other diagnostic modalities is that it can be used as a one-stop examination.[35] Whole body FDG-PET/CT mammography protocol may be used for staging breast cancer in a single session.[36] FDG-PET/CT is also a valuable modality for follow-up of patients who have elevated levels of tumor markers.[37]

FDG-PET–DYNAMIC CONTRAST-ENHANCED CT

The process of malignant transformation is complex, involving many alterations in the metabolic and functional status of tumor cells and is unique to every cancer. Combined FDG-PET/CT has higher sensitivity and specificity than separate FDG-PET and CT in evaluating various cancers.

RATIONALE FOR FDG-PET/ CONTRAST-ENHANCED CT

FDG-PET and FDG-PET/CT heavily rely on the metabolic activity of FDG detected with its FDG-PET component. The perfusion component of CT using intravenous iodinated contrast material is largely unexplored. Moreover, CECT is often performed for staging purposes. Therefore, the authors conceptualized simultaneous acquisition of PET and CECT data to enhance the effect of existing PET/CT.

FDG-PET/CONTRAST-ENHANCED CT PERFUSION

Perfusion imaging is a functional study that can quantify tumor angiogenesis, blood perfusion, and vascular permeability.[38] It can also evaluate the early effects of therapeutic interventions in malignant solid tumors. The availability of rapid imaging with MDCT systems and robust computing software has made CT perfusion imaging a reality. Dynamic CECT (DCECT) can measure the regional blood flow and volume along with mean transit time of blood through the capillaries. Therefore, combined FDG-PET/DCECT can assess not only glucose metabolism of tumors but also tumor vascularity. Both of these parameters can be used to differentiate between malignant and benign tumors, evaluate tumor aggressiveness, determine tumor response to therapy and occult residual tumors, and delineate the tumor during radiotherapy planning. Therefore, FDG-PET/ DCECT can improve the diagnosis, prognosis, treatment selection, and therapy monitoring of various cancers.[39]

VALIDATION AND REPRODUCIBILITY OF FDG-PET/CONTRAST-ENHANCED CT

CT perfusion methods have been validated in humans using stable xenon washout techniques.[40–42] Literature suggests an increasing role of CT perfusion in evaluating solitary pulmonary nodules, colorectal carcinoma, hepatocellular carcinoma, and nasopharyngeal carcinoma. Reproducibility studies show good correlation for perfusion CT measurements in colorectal carcinoma, lung cancer, and hepatocellular carcinoma.[43–48]

Goh and colleagues[48] found that perfusion CT values were reproducible and also noted that variability was less for tumors than for skeletal muscle. Only a few published studies use DCECT perfusion and PET data. Further studies recruiting larger numbers of patients would validate the FDG-PET/ DCECT technique. Baseline reproducibility studies may be needed to ensure the accuracy of simultaneous perfusion measurements using DCECT with PET.

CURRENT APPLICATIONS

Akashi-Tanaka and colleagues[49] recently concluded that all breast cancers could be distinguished from normal mammary glands based on the perfusion value, which was measured using a 256-row MDCT scanner. The extent of cancer depicted on perfusion images showed excellent agreement with the pathology findings for invasive ductal carcinoma and ductal carcinoma in situ. These results suggest that volume perfusion imaging may be useful for depicting the extent of breast cancer, although further study is needed to determine its clinical relevance.

DCECT imaging has shown that CT perfusion data closely correlate with tumor angiogenesis and reflect microvessel density measurement and vascular endothelial growth factor expression in solitary pulmonary nodules.[50] Goh and colleagues[51] showed that tumor blood flow differed significantly between disease-free individuals and patients who had metastatic colorectal cancer.

Accurate and precise measurement of hepatic arterial blood flow is possible with DCECT. In patients who have hepatocellular carcinoma and cirrhosis, in whom FDG-PET has a limited role, CT perfusion data from FDG-PET/DCECT can play an important role in providing quantitative information about tumor-related angiogenesis.[52]

Zhou and colleagues[53] reported that perfusion parameters (blood flow, blood volume), mean transit time, and permeability surface measured with perfusion CT are significantly altered in nasopharyngeal cancer. Metabolic flow relationships of tumors have been shown using different FDG-PET tracers.[54–56] However, H2 15O is not easily available or routinely used in clinical practice, and also requires an onsite cyclotron.

Mankoff and colleagues[54] showed the value of combining FDG metabolic FDG-PET data with perfusion data obtained using H2 15O in locally advanced breast cancer over the course of neoadjuvant chemotherapy. The authors concluded that tumor metabolic and perfusion changes in locally advanced breast cancer can differentiate responders and nonresponders. Patients who had no significant decline in tumor perfusion after 2 months of therapy had poorer disease-free and overall survival.

In another study, the same group compared tumor blood flow and glucose metabolism with clinical and pathologic parameters and with response to chemotherapy in patients who had locally advanced breast cancer.[55] The tumor blood flow and glucose metabolism were significantly higher in patients who had tumors than in those who had normal breasts.

In another study, Hentschel and colleagues[56] also found significantly higher perfusion and glucose metabolism in tumors than in normal breast tissue. Both studies showed a positive correlation between glucose metabolism detected with FDG and tumor blood flow.

In a recently published study, Groves and colleagues[57] found a good correlation between metabolic components of FDG-PET and blood flow measured with DCECT in evaluating primary breast cancer. The authors found a significant correlation with standard uptake value when perfusion was normalized to cardiac output. The perfusion and metabolic components of the hybrid FDG-PET/CT scanner may be complementary, as shown by Groves and colleagues,[57] and further study is required to standardize the technique and to establish its validity. The importance of tissue perfusion and metabolic coupling is also evident in lung cancer and head and neck squamous cell carcinomas, and may provide additional diagnostic information in patients undergoing FDG-PET/CT studies.[58,59] FDG-PET/CT can improve staging and alter therapeutic options in patients suspected to have breast cancer recurrence and distant metastatic disease, primarily by demonstrating local or distant nodal involvement occult at other imaging studies. The added value of FDG-PET/CT over other diagnostic modalities is mainly expressed by the fact that a noninvasive whole-body evaluation is possible in a single examination.[60] Dirisamer and colleagues[35] studied the possibility of diagnostic CECT and FDG-PET in a one-step investigation to determine whether diagnostic FDG-PET/CT provides more information than FDG-PET or CECT alone for restaging patients who have suspected breast cancer recurrence. FDG-PET, CT, and FDG-PET/CT had a sensitivity and specificity for lesion detection of 84%, 66%, and 93%, and 100%, 92%, and 100%, respectively.[35]

FUTURE APPLICATIONS

With functional imaging set to heavily supplant, if not completely replace, many traditional biochemical and physiologic tests in the near future, the scope of imaging is bound to expand into new spheres of influence. In keeping with this realistic anticipation, the combined technique of FDG-PET and DCECT may open up a new area of breast cancer research. Dynamic MRI has been commonly used to measure perfusion of various tumors, with implications in the diagnosis, staging, and evaluation of treatment response of breast cancer.[60]

Semple and colleagues[61] investigated the relationship between vascular and metabolic characteristics of breast tumor using dynamic contrast-enhanced MRI and FDG-PET imaging. The authors found a good correlation between tumor vascularity and metabolism. Another study comparing dynamic MRI and FDG-PET showed almost identical the results concerning the diagnosis of primary breast lesions.[62] MRI and FDG-PET fusion is possible and prone mammography FDG-PET acquisition improves the ability to fuse MRI with FDG-PET.[63] Compared with DCECT, dynamic MRI has certain advantages, such as no immediate reaction to intravenous contrast material and no radiation exposure to the patient.

The combination of DWI and DCE-MRI could produce high diagnostic accuracy for characterizing enhanced mass on breast MRI.[64] Sensitivity encoding DWI may provide more detailed information about lesions, including tumor cellularity, which is difficult to obtain with conventional techniques.[65] However, DWI seems to be insensitive for determining the antiangiogenic treatment response in osteolytic breast cancer.[66] The DWI image can be inverted to get a PET-like image.

In this era of rapidly changing technology, FDG-PET/MRI-DWI fusion images may soon be available for routine clinical use. Once the this occurs, it will be interesting to see what will be the role of FDG-PET/DCECT.

LIMITATIONS

Tumor perfusion data obtained with FDG-PET/ DCECT will have certain limitations because the software calculating these data is based on certain assumptions. The perfusion parameter result from time–contrast enhancement curves within an arterial input is uniform. However, contrast enhancement within tumor tissue is not uniform. Moreover, contrast used for this technique is not ideal to measure correct perfusion and is certainly inferior to 15O perfusion data. The role in hypoxic tumor cells is also uncertain. Similar to other tests, this technique will also provide false-negative and -positive results under certain conditions. Slow growing and well-differentiated histologic subtypes of tumors, such as tubular, in situ, and lobular carcinomas, show near-normal or a mild increase in perfusion, and therefore false-negative results will be noted. Similarly, false-positive results are likely to occur in patients who have a history of recent surgery, chemotherapy, and radiotherapy, because these conditions cause increased perfusion.

SUMMARY

Breast cancer is a complex disease and molecular imaging may contribute to better management through providing new insight for early detection. FDG-PET/CT has made great strides as a functional anatomic technique and recently gained attention in the diagnosis, staging, and follow-up of breast cancer. FDG-PET and CT complement each other's strengths in integrated FDG-PET/CT. One-stop-shop whole-body FDG-PET/CT coupled with integrated FDG-PET/CT mammography has also been advocated.

FDG-PET is a highly sensitive modality for depicting the whole-body distribution of positron-emitting biomarkers indicating tumor metabolic activity. However, conventional FDG-PET imaging is lacking detailed anatomic information to precisely localize pathologic findings. CECT imaging can readily provide the required morphologic data, and CT perfusion can assess the tumor neovascularity. Thus, integrated FDG-PET/DCECT represents an efficient tool for whole-body staging and functional assessment within one examination. Because of developments in system technology, FDG-PET/CT devices are continually gaining spatial resolution and imaging speed.

Whole-body imaging from the head to the upper thighs is accomplished in less than 20 minutes, promoting FDG-PET/DCECT as the preferred imaging modality for workup of the most common tumor entities and some of the rare malignancies. FDG-PET/MRI fusion is also feasible and may assist in localizing lesions detected on either study. A more extensive study is underway to confirm the value of this fusion technique.

FDG-PET/MRI-DWI fusion imaging is also expected in the near future. This combined method may further widen the field of breast cancer imaging and improve patient care. Ongoing research; new tracers other than FDG, such as fluorine-18; and new instruments, such as FDG-PET/CT and positron emission mammography, are likely to improve patient care. FDG-PET/CT should be used in addition to conventional radiologic methods. Hybrid FDG-PET/CECT imaging should be used in the appropriate clinical setting to diagnose, stage, and detect recurrence of breast cancer. In conclusion, combined FDG-PET/DCECT imaging techniques are still evolving and methods of image analysis remain variable and nonstandard. The perfusion data obtained with DCECT seem promising and likely to have some incremental value over structural and metabolic data provided by FDG-PET/CT. The results of initial published studies using perfusion data are encouraging. However, further studies recruiting larger numbers of patients would define the role of FDG-PET/DCECT and its future indications in the management of breast cancer.

REFERENCES

1. National Cancer Institute. Available at: http://www.cancer.gov/cancertopics/types/breast. Accessed May 17, 2009.
2. Shimizu C, Ando M, Kouno T, et al. Current trends and controversies over pre-operative chemotherapy for women with operable breast cancer. Jpn J Clin Oncol 2007;37(1):1–8.
3. Polsky D, Mandelblatt JS, Weeks JC, et al. Economic evaluation of breast cancer treatment: considering the value of patient choice. J Clin Oncol 2003; 21(6):1139–46.
4. Wolff AC, Davidson NE. Early operable breast cancer. Curr Treat Options Oncol 2000;1:210–20.
5. Vlastos G, Mirza NQ, Meric F, et al. Breast conservation therapy as a treatment option for the elderly. The M.D. Anderson experience. Cancer 2001;92(5): 1092–100.
6. Anderssona, Awadab A, Barrett-Leec P, et al. European oncologists' preferences for the management of breast cancer: case presentations and expert commentary. Breast 2008;17(Suppl 2):S1–12.
7. Buscombe JR, Holloway B, Roche N, et al. Position of nuclear medicine modalities in the diagnostic work-up of breast cancer. Q J Nucl Med Mol Imaging 2004;48(2):109–18.
8. The JS, Schilling KJ, Hoffmeister JW, et al. Detection of breast cancer with full-field digital mammography and computer-aided detection. AJR Am J Roentgenol 2009;192(2):337–40.

9. Scheidhauer K, Walter C, Seemann MD. FDG PET and other imaging modalities in the primary diagnosis of suspicious breast lesions. Eur J Nucl Med Mol Imaging 2004;31(Suppl 1):S70–9.

10. Lo GG, Ai V, Chan JK, et al. Diffusion-weighted magnetic resonance imaging of breast lesions: first experiences at 3 T. J Comput Assist Tomogr 2009; 33(1):63–9.

11. Wang L, Yao Q, Wang J, et al. MRI and hybrid PET/CT for monitoring tumour metastasis in a metastatic breast cancer model in rabbit. Nucl Med Commun 2008;29(2):137–43.

12. Rosen EL, Eubank WB, Mankoff DA. FDG PET, PET/CT, and breast cancer imaging. Radiographics 2007;27(Suppl 1):S215–29.

13. Wu D, Gambhir SS. Positron emission tomography in diagnosis and management of invasive breast cancer: current status and future perspectives. Clin Breast Cancer 2003;4(Suppl 1):S55–63.

14. Heinisch M, Gallowitsch HJ, Mikosch P, et al. Comparison of FDG-PET and dynamic contrast-enhanced MRI in the evaluation of suggestive breast lesions. Breast 2003;12(1):17–22.

15. Basu S, Mavi A, Cermik T, et al. Implications of standardized uptake value measurements of the primary lesions in proven cases of breast carcinoma with different degree of disease burden at diagnosis: does 2-deoxy-2-[F-18]fluoro-D-glucose-positron emission tomography predict tumor biology? Mol Imaging Biol 2008;10:62–6.

16. Kumar R, Das CJ. Hybrid PET-dynamic CECT in the management of breast cancer. Eur J Nucl Med Mol Imaging 2009;36(3):413–5.

17. Chae BJ, Chae BJ, Bae JS, et al. Positron emission tomography-computed tomography in the detection of axillary lymph node metastasis in patients with early stage breast cancer. Jpn J Clin Oncol 2009; 39(5):284–9.

18. Mahner S, Schirrmacher S, Brenner W, et al. Comparison between positron emission tomography using 2-[fluorine-18]fluoro-2-deoxy-D-glucose, conventional imaging and computed tomography for staging of breast cancer. Ann Oncol 2008;19(7):1249–54.

19. Gallowitsch HJ, Kresnik E, Gasser J, et al. F-18 fluorodeoxyglucose positron-emission tomography in the diagnosis of tumor recurrence and metastases in the follow-up of patients with breast carcinoma: a comparison to conventional imaging. Invest Radiol 2003;38(5):250–6.

20. Lind P, Igerc I, Beyer T, et al. Advantages and limitations of FDG PET in the follow-up of breast cancer. Eur J Nucl Med Mol Imaging 2004;31(Suppl 1): S125–34.

21. Blodgett TM, Meltzer CC, Townsend DW. PET/CT: form and function. Radiology 2007;242(2):360–85.

22. Veit-Haibach P, Antoch G, Beyer T, et al. FDG-PET/CT in restaging of patients with recurrent breast cancer: possible impact on staging and therapy. Br J Radiol 2007;80(955):508–15.

23. Zytoon AA, Murakami K, El-Kholy MR, et al. Dual time point FDG-PET/CT imaging. Potential tool for diagnosis of breast cancer. Clin Radiol 2008; 63(11):1213–27.

24. Lovrics PJ, Chen V, Coates G, et al. A prospective evaluation of positron emission tomography scanning, sentinel lymph node biopsy, and standard axillary dissection for axillary staging in patients with early stage breast cancer. Ann Surg Oncol 2004; 11(9):846–53.

25. Fuster D, Duch J, Paredes P, et al. Preoperative staging of large primary breast cancer with [18F]fluorodeoxyglucose positron emission tomography/computed tomography compared with conventional imaging procedures. J Clin Oncol 2008;26(29): 4746–51.

26. Taira N, Ohsumi S, Takabatake D, et al. Determination of indication for sentinel lymph node biopsy in clinical node-negative breast cancer using preoperative 18F-fluorodeoxyglucose positron emission tomography/computed tomography fusion imaging. Jpn J Clin Oncol 2009;39(1):16–21.

27. Heusner TA, Hahn S, Hamami ME, et al. Incidental head and neck (18)F-FDG uptake on PET/CT without corresponding morphological lesion: early predictor of cancer development? Eur J Nucl Med Mol Imaging 2009;36(9):1397–406.

28. Kim J, Lee J, Chang E, et al. Selective sentinel node plus additional non-sentinel node biopsy based on an FDG-PET/CT Scan in early breast cancer patients: single institutional experience. World J Surg 2009;33(5):943–9.

29. Ueda S, Tsuda H, Asakawa H, et al. Utility of 18F-fluorodeoxyglucose emission tomography/computed tomography fusion imaging (18F-FDG PET/CT) in combination with ultrasonography for axillary staging in primary breast cancer. BMC Cancer 2008;8:165.

30. Pons F, Duch J, Fuster D. Breast cancer therapy: the role of PET-CT in decision making. Q J Nucl Med Mol Imaging 2009;53(2):210–28.

31. Carkaci S, Macapinlac HA, Cristofanilli M, et al. Retrospective study of 18F-FDG PET/CT in the diagnosis of inflammatory breast cancer: preliminary data. J Nucl Med 2009;50:231–8.

32. Fueger BJ, Weber WA, Quon A, et al. Performance of 2-deoxy-2-[F-18]fluoro-D-glucose positron emission tomography and integrated PET/CT in restaged breast cancer patients. Mol Imaging Biol 2005;7(5): 369–76.

33. Kumar A, Kumar R, Seenu V, et al. The role of 18F-FDG PET/CT in evaluation of early response to neoadjuvant chemotherapy in patients with locally advanced breast cancer. Eur Radiol 2009;19(6):1347–67.

34. Li D, Yao Q, Li L, et al. Correlation between hybrid 18F-FDG PET/CT and apoptosis induced by

neoadjuvant chemotherapy in breast cancer. Cancer Biol Ther 2007;6(9):1442–8.

35. Dirisamer A, Halpern BS, Flöry D, et al. Integrated contrast-enhanced diagnostic whole-body PET/CT as a first-line restaging modality in patients with suspected metastatic recurrence of breast cancer. Eur J Radiol 2009 [Epub ahead of print].

36. Heusner TA, Kuemmel S, Umutlu L, et al. Breast cancer staging in a single session: whole-body PET/CT mammography. J Nucl Med 2008;49(8): 1215–22.

37. Haug AR, Schmidt GP, Klingenstein A, et al. F-18-fluoro-2-deoxyglucose positron emission tomography/computed tomography in the follow-up of breast cancer with elevated levels of tumor markers. J Comput Assist Tomogr 2007;31(4):629–34.

38. Sahani DV, Kalva SP, Hamberg LM, et al. Assessing tumor perfusion and treatment response in rectal cancer with multisection CT: initial observations. Radiology 2005;234(3):785–92.

39. Willett CG, Boucher Y, di Tomaso E, et al. Direct evidence that the VEGF-specific antibody bevacizumab has antivascular effects in human rectal cancer. Nat Med 2004;10(2):145–7.

40. Cenic A, Nabavi DG, Craen RA, et al. Dynamic CT measurement of cerebral blood flow: a validation study. AJNR Am J Neuroradiol 1999;20(1):63–73.

41. Gobbel GT, Cann CE, Fike JR. Comparison of xenon-enhanced CT with ultrafast CT for measurement of regional cerebral blood flow. AJNR Am J Neuroradiol 1993;14(3):543–50.

42. Gobbel GT, Cann CE, Iwamoto HS, et al. Measurement of regional cerebral blood flow in the dog using ultrafast computed tomography. Experimental validation. Stroke 1991;22(6):772–9.

43. Sahani DV, Holalkere NS, Mueller PR, et al. Advanced hepatocellular carcinoma: CT perfusion of liver and tumor tissue—initial experience. Radiology 2007;243(3):736–43.

44. Goh V, Halligan S, Hugill JA, et al. Quantitative assessment of colorectal cancer perfusion using MDCT: inter- and intraobserver agreement. AJR Am J Roentgenol 2005;185(1):225–31.

45. Cenic A, Nabavi DG, Craen RA, et al. A CT method to measure hemodynamics in brain tumors: validation and application of cerebral blood flow maps. AJNR Am J Neuroradiol 2000;21(3):462–70.

46. Gillard JH, Antoun NM, Burnet NG, et al. Reproducibility of quantitative CT perfusion imaging. Br J Radiol 2001;74(882):552–5.

47. Nabavi DG, Cenic A, Dool J, et al. Quantitative assessment of cerebral hemodynamics using CT: stability, accuracy, and precision studies in dogs. J Comput Assist Tomogr 1999;23(4):506–15.

48. Goh V, Halligan S, Hugill JA, et al. Quantitative assessment of tissue perfusion using MDCT: comparison of colorectal cancer and skeletal muscle measurement reproducibility. AJR Am J Roentgenol 2006;187(1):164–9.

49. Akashi-Tanaka S, Shien T, Tsukagoshi S, et al. Whole-breast volume perfusion images using 256-row multislice computed tomography: visualization of lesions with ductal spread. Breast Cancer 2009; 16:62–7.

50. Ma SH, Le HB, Jia BH, et al. Peripheral pulmonary nodules: relationship between multi-slice spiral CT perfusion imaging and tumour angiogenesis and VEGF expression. BMC Cancer 2008;8:186.

51. Goh V, Halligan S, Wellsted DM, et al. Can perfusion CT assessment of primary colorectal adenocarcinoma blood flow at staging predict for subsequent metastatic disease? A pilot study. Eur Radiol 2009; 19(1):79–89.

52. Ippolito D, Sironi S, Pozzi M, et al. Hepatocellular carcinoma in cirrhotic liver disease: functional computed tomography with perfusion imaging in the assessment of tumour vascularization. Acad Radiol 2008;15:919–27.

53. Zhou Z, Wu J, Han M, et al. MSCT perfusion analysis of nasopharyngeal cancer. Lin Chung Er Bi Yan Hou Tou Jing Wai Ke Za Zhi 2008;22:150–2.

54. Mankoff DA, Dunnwald LK, Gralow JR, et al. Changes in blood flow and metabolism in locally advanced breast cancer treated with neoadjuvant chemotherapy. J Nucl Med 2003;44:1806–14.

55. Mankoff DA, Dunnwald LK, Gralow JR, et al. Blood flow and metabolism in locally advanced breast cancer: relationship to response to therapy. J Nucl Med 2002;43:500–9.

56. Hentschel M, Paulus T, Mix M, et al. Analysis of blood flow and glucose metabolism in mammary carcinomas and normal breast: a H2(15)O PET and 18F-FDG PET study. Nucl Med Commun 2007;28: 789–97.

57. Groves AM, Wishart GC, Shastry M, et al. Metabolic-flow relationships in primary breast cancer: feasibility of combined PET/dynamic contrast-enhanced CT. Eur J Nucl Med Mol Imaging 2009;36(3):416–21.

58. Miles KA, Griffiths MR, Keith CJ. Blood flow-metabolic relationships are dependent on tumour size in non-small cell lung cancer: a study using quantitative contrast-enhanced computer tomography and positron emission tomography. Eur J Nucl Med Mol Imaging 2006;33:22–8.

59. Bisdas S, Spicer K, Rumboldt Z. Whole-tumour perfusion CT parameters and glucose metabolism measurements in head and neck squamous cell carcinomas: a pilot study using combined positron emission tomography/CT imaging. AJNR Am J Neuroradiol 2008;29:1376–81.

60. Hayes C, Padhani AR, Leach MO. Assessing changes in tumour vascular function using dynamic contrast-enhanced magnetic resonance imaging. NMR Biomed 2002;15:154–63.

61. Semple SI, Gilbert FJ, Redpath TW, et al. The relationship between vascular and metabolic characteristics of primary breast tumours. Eur Radiol 2004;14:
2038–45.

62. Brix G, Henze M, Knopp MV, et al. Comparison of
pharmacokinetic MRI and [18F] fluorodeoxyglucose
PET in the diagnosis of breast cancer: initial experience. Eur Radiol 2001;11:2058–70.

63. Moy L, Noz ME, Maguire GQ Jr, et al. Prone mamm-
moPET acquisition improves the ability to fuse MRI
and PET breast scans. Clin Nucl Med 2007;32:
194–8.

64. Yabuuchi H, Matsuo Y, Okafuji T, et al. Enhanced
mass on contrast-enhanced breast MR imaging:
lesion characterization using combination of
dynamic contrast-enhanced and diffusion-weighted
MR images. J Magn Reson Imaging 2008;28(5):
1157–65.

65. Kuroki Y, Nasu K, Kuroki S, et al. Diffusion-weighted
imaging of breast cancer with the sensitivity encoding technique: analysis of the apparent diffusion
coefficient value. Magn Reson Med Sci 2004;3(2):
79–85.

66. Bäuerle T, Bartling S, Berger M, et al. Imaging antiangiogenic treatment response with DCE-VCT,
DCE-MRI and DWI in an animal model of breast
cancer bone metastasis. Eur J Radiol 2008 [Epub
ahead of print].

The Role of Lymphatic Mapping and Sentinel Lymph Node Biopsy in the Staging of Breast Cancer

Robert E. Roses, MD[a], Rakesh Kumar, MD[b],
Abass Alavi, MD, MD (Hon), PhD (Hon), DSc (Hon)[c],
Brian J. Czerniecki, MD, PhD[a,b,*]

KEYWORDS

- Sentinel lymph node biopsy • Breast cancer
- Positron emission tomography (PET) • Staging

BACKGROUND

The status of the axillary lymph nodes (i.e., the presence or absence of nodal metastases) is the most significant prognostic factor in patients with cancer of the breast. More than any other factor, axillary nodal metastases predict poorer survival and a higher likelihood of disease recurrence.[1] Moreover, the number of metastatic axillary nodes,[1–3] the size of metastases,[4,5] and extension of metastases beyond the nodal capsule[6] all portend poorer survival. No clinical or radiographic approach has proven reliable in identifying nodal metastases in patients with invasive breast cancer. Although physical examination can often identify the presence of gross axillary disease, the frequencies of false-negative and false-positive examination findings are high. A variety of features of a primary tumor are associated with an increased likelihood of nodal disease. Although larger tumor size, lymphatic or vascular invasion, and HER-2/neu overexpression are all associated with a high risk of nodal metastases in some series,[7–9] none has displaced pathologic assessment of the axillary nodes as an effective staging technique. Likewise, mammography, sonography, MRI, and positron emission tomography (PET)[10–13] have emerged as useful adjuncts but have not supplanted surgical staging.

Until the 1990s, axillary dissection represented the preferred approach for nodal staging and it remains an important component of the treatment of invasive breast cancer. Although generally well tolerated, this procedure is associated with a risk of postoperative pain, parasthesias, and lymphedema. Moreover, only those patients with axillary nodal metastases derive a potential therapeutic benefit from lymphadenectomy. In the late 1960s, Cabanas[14] introduced the idea that a cutaneous lesion, in this case a penile carcinoma, would initially drain to a specific lymph node—the sentinel node. Biopsy of the sentinel node could be used to predict the presence of nonsentinel nodal metastases. The technique of sentinel node biopsy was subsequently refined and applied to the management of cutaneous melanoma by Morton. In a single-center and then a multicenter trial, Morton and colleagues demonstrated that melanoma could be reliably staged using this technique with negligible rates of false-positive results and low rates of false-negative results (ie, cases in which

[a] Department of Surgery, University of Pennsylvania School of Medicine, 4 Silverstein, 3400 Spruce Street, Philadelphia, PA 19104, USA
[b] Department of Nuclear Medicine, All India Institute of Medical Sciences, New Delhi, India
[c] Department Section, Radiology, University of Pennsylvania School of Medicine, Philadelphia, PA, USA
* Corresponding author. Department of Surgery, University of Pennsylvania School of Medicine, 4 Silverstein, 3400 Spruce Street, Philadelphia, PA 19104, USA.
E-mail address: brian.czerniecki@uphs.upenn.edu (B.J. Czerniecki).

PET Clin 4 (2009) 265–276
doi:10.1016/j.cpet.2009.09.004

a sentinel node was negative but metastases were identified in nonsentinel nodes).[15,16] Shortly after the introduction of sentinel lymph node biopsy in the management of cutaneous melanoma, Giuliano and colleagues[17] and Krag and colleagues[18] applied similar approaches to the staging of breast cancer. Sentinel lymph node biopsy for the staging of invasive breast cancer has subsequently been validated with reported rates of successful of sentinel lymph node identification exceeding 95%. Rates of false-positive results range from 0 to 13% in series in which sentinel lymph node biopsy is followed by completion axillary dissection.[19]

MECHANISMS OF SENTINEL NODE UPTAKE

Although sentinel lymph node biopsy has been widely accepted for the staging of cutaneous melanoma and breast cancer, some mechanistic aspects of the procedure remain poorly understood. Although the distribution of radiolabeled tracer in the lymphatics and regional nodes has often been attributed to passive processes influenced mainly by particle size, increasingly it has become apparent that active mechanisms of tracer distribution also play a role.[20,21] When administered into the interstitium of the breast, radioisotope-labeled colloids passively transit to the draining lymph node basin. After particles enter the lymphatics and travel to nodes, they may be taken up by antigen presenting cells within sentinel nodes by macropinocytosis.[16] This immunologically determined uptake, to some extent, defines the sentinel nodes—those nodes whose role it is to actively survey drainage from the tumor site.

As discussed previously, the range of particle sizes in a given radioactive colloid preparation is a major determinant of the kinetics of the passive distribution of tracer. Smaller particles reach the draining lymph node basin and proceed to higher-echelon nodes more rapidly than do larger particles. By extension, the rapidity with which the contribution of active uptake overtakes that of passive distribution also depends on the size of tracer particles. Tracer preparations containing larger particles label a greater proportion of nodes that are not immunologically determined at earlier time points. Conversely, smaller particle preparations transit to the nodes more readily where they may be actively taken up.[21] The interaction between these active and passive mechanisms of distribution may have implications for tracer selection and timing of injection (discussed later).

INDICATIONS FOR SENTINEL LYMPH NODE BIOPSY
Invasive Breast Cancer

Patients with invasive breast cancer who can safely undergo surgery benefit from lymph node staging. Exceptions include patients with axillary lymphadenopathy suspicious for metastatic disease and patients who have had prior breast or chest wall irradiation, which may disrupt the lymphatics and preclude accurate lymphatic mapping. Such patients should forgo sentinel lymph node biopsy in favor of axillary dissection. Conversely, elderly patients or those with significant comorbidities, with favorable stage I tumors, may forgo sentinel lymph node biopsy. This includes patients with small (<1 cm), well-differentiated (eg, colloid and tubular carcinomas) tumors, which are rarely associated with lymph node metastases.[22–24]

Ductal Carcinoma in Situ

Histologic assessment of the axilla has not generally been advocated for patients with predominantly intraductal disease with or without microinvasion. Although patients with in situ breast cancers should not, theoretically, have nodal metastases, occult invasive foci are present in 10% to 30% of such patients. Sentinel lymph node biopsy is, therefore, considered in patients with multicentric or broad areas of high-grade ductal carcinoma in situ (DCIS) and those with DCIS undergoing total mastectomy, which precludes subsequent nodal staging without axillary dissection. Additionally, several histologic features of DCIS have been associated with the presence of occult invasive disease and, therefore, constitute relative indications for lymph node staging. These include high nuclear grade, the presence of comedo necrosis, and the presence of a palpable or radiographic mass.[25,26] We have demonstrated a strong association between HER-2/neu overexpression in DCIS and the presence of associated invasive foci.[27] Patients with HER-2/neu positive DCIS may be at increased risk of harboring invasive disease and benefit from sentinel lymph node biopsy.

TECHNICAL CONSIDERATIONS

Sentinel node biopsy requires the coordination of nuclear medicine specialists, surgeons, and pathologists. Lymphoscintigraphy can be performed on the day before, or on the day of, surgery. Technetium-99m (99mTc)–sulfur colloid (SC) or an alternative mapping agent is injected into the peritumoral, intratumoral, or subareolar breast tissue or into the dermis overlying the tumor. At some institutions, patients are then imaged using a large field-of-view gamma camera with high-resolution collimator. Static images can be taken at serial intervals after the injection of radiotracer. After localization of the tracer, antero-posterior and lateral images are taken to document the site of the radiographically identified draining lymph nodes. All such lymph nodes are marked on the overlying skin with indelible ink. Patients are then transported to an operating room.

Intraoperatively, Lymphazurin blue or an alternative dye is injected into at one of the sites (described previously). In general, the sentinel lymph node procedure is performed before (re)-excision of the breast tumor. After administration of anesthesia, positioning of the patient on the operating table, and sterile preparation of the surgical site, a skin incision is made directly over the hottest axillary site (as identified by a gamma detecting probe). Dissection is performed to identify all blue lymphatics and blue nodes. Blue nodes are removed. Additional dissection to identify isotope-positive nodes is guided by the gamma detecting probe. Isotope-positive nodes are defined as nodes with counts at least three times background or 10 times that of ex vivo fat. Isotope-positive nodes are removed until the background axillary counts are less than 10% that of the hottest node removed.[28]

The sentinel lymph nodes are formalin fixed, paraffin embedded, and evaluated with hematoxylin-eosin stain, and, at some centers, immunohistochemistry. A micrometastasis is defined as a tumor deposit of less than 2.0 mm. A metastasis of 2.0 mm or greater is considered to be a macrometastasis. The presence or absence of isolated tumor cells is also noted. If multiple tumor deposits are present in the sentinel lymph node, the sum of the tumor deposits is used to classify the metastasis as micro- or macrometastasis.[29]

CHOICE OF MAPPING AGENT
Radiolabeled Tracers

Different radiolabeled tracers have been evaluated for use in sentinel lymph node biopsy. Early studies by Krag and colleagues[30] used radiolabeled 99mTc-SC and a handheld gamma probe for detection. This technique was associated with a sentinel node identification rate of 98% and a false-negative rate of 11%. The use of a variety of radiolabeled tracers with different ranges of particle sizes has subsequently been explored. As discussed previously, particle size is an important determinant of the kinetics of tracer distribution; smaller particles more rapidly concentrate in the nodal basin and progress to higher-echelon nodes than do larger particles. 99mTc-SC, unfiltered (with particles ranging from 15 to 5000 nm) or filtered, is the most commonly used agent in the United States. Although filtered preparations are widely used, there are some data to suggest that unfiltered preparations are associated with higher rates of sentinel node identification.[31] Outside of the United States, 99mTc-nanocolloid human serum albumin (with particles between 4 and 100 nm) and 99mTc-antimony trisulfide (3 to 30 nm) are used more frequently.[32] More recently, several mannose-binding agents have been developed for sentinel lymph node imaging.[33–36] These include 99mTc-diethylenetriaminepentaacetic acid–mannosyl polymer[33] and 99mTc-neomannosyl human serum albumin.[35] Such agents have the potential advantages of rapid clearance from the injection site (owing to small particle size) coupled with better retention in sentinel nodes (owing to mannose receptor binding). Preclinical and early clinical data suggest promising properties of these agents.

Dyes

Giuliano and colleagues[37] used isosulfan blue dye alone in their early studies and reported sentinel node identification rates similar to those achieved with radioisotope but with a lower false-negative rate. A distinct disadvantage of isosulfan blue dye is the small associated risk (1% to 3%) of anaphylaxis or more mild allergic reactions.[38,39] Some data suggest that methylene blue is a less expensive, similarly reliable alternative and is associated with a lower risk of allergic reactions.[40] Skin necrosis and dermolysis are associated with subcutaneous methylene blue dye injection. Most centers have adopted dual injection with radioisotope and blue dye, an approach associated with the highest rates of sentinel node identification. In a prospective, multicenter analysis of 3961 patients by Chagpar and colleagues,[41] the combination of radioactive colloid injection plus blue dye was compared with blue dye or radioactive colloid alone. Sentinel lymph node identification rates were significantly higher when the two techniques were combined than with injection of radioactive colloid or the use of blue dye alone (P<.001). The false-negative rates were similar for all techniques. In a second study of 4131 patients who underwent sentinel lymph node biopsy from the same group, the use of blue dye alone independently predicted a higher rate of failure in identifying sentinel nodes (odds ratio 0.389, $P<.001$).[42]

ROUTE OF INJECTION

The accuracy of sentinel lymph node biopsy when tracer or blue dye is injected at different sites, including the peritumoral breast parenchyma, the tumor itself, the peritumoral dermis or subdermis, and the subareolar lymphatic plexus, has been explored in several studies. Most early studies used the peritumoral route.[30,37] This approach has several disadvantages: (1) in some cases, the integrity of the lymphatic drainage in the peritumoral lymphatics may be compromised by tumor infiltration leading to poorer lymphatic mapping; (2) in patients with nonpalpable tumors, this method requires the use of imaging to guide injection; and (3) in patients with tumors closer to the axilla (ie, upper outer quadrant masses), peritumoral injection may lead to shine-through of radioactivity from the breast into the axilla, and detection of this radioactivity with the gamma probe can undermine efforts to identify the sentinel node. For these reasons, other approaches have been explored. Injection into, or directly under, the skin overlying the tumor theoretically take advantage of the reliably rich lymphatic supply at these sites and are advocated by some groups.[43,44]

Most of the lymphatics of the breast parenchyma drain through the subareolar lymphatic plexus of Sappey. Injection directly into the subareolar space allows for identification of sentinel nodes in most cases. The authors and other investigators have demonstrated that this approach identifies similar sentinel nodes to those identified after peritumoral injection.[29,41,45,46] This approach has several advantages, including its ready application in cases where the primary tumor is nonpalpable. Moreover, shine-through of radioactivity from the breast to the axilla is virtually eliminated using this approach, irrespective of the site of the primary tumor. A disadvantage of this approach is the blue staining of the breast, which may persist for as long as several months. Additionally, some investigators have raised the concern that lymphatic mapping may be misleading in those cases in which the tumor drains to internal mammary of supraclavicular nodes.[47] In a study comparing peritumoral and subareolar injection of radiotracer, the authors identified internal mammary nodes more frequently with peritumoral compared with subareolar injection of radiotracer.[29] The clinical significance, however, of identifying internal mammary

nodal drainage or metastases remains controversial.[48–50]

TIMING OF RADIOISOTOPE INJECTION AND LYMPHOSCINTIGRAPHY

At many centers, injection with radioisotope is followed by a lymphoscintigram to aid in identification of the sentinel node. Such imaging is typically performed beginning 20 minutes or more after injection and consists of anterior and lateral views. The lymphoscintigram may be serially repeated until the primary draining nodal basin is identified and adequate tracer uptake is confirmed. In patients with melanoma, the argument for preoperative lymphoscintigraphy is compelling, given the variability of the lymphatic drainage from many cutaneous sites. Imaging in these patients is sometimes invaluable in planning sentinel node biopsy. In patients with breast cancer, lymphoscintigraphy may be of use in identifying those patients with sentinel internal mammary or supraclavicular nodes. These patients, however, represent a small minority of all patients with breast cancer, and the clinical significance of detecting such drainage patterns remains unclear.[48–50] Some investigators have, therefore, questioned the need for preoperative lymphoscintigraphy. McMasters and colleagues[51] compared rates of sentinel node identification, false-negative results, and number of sentinel node identification in 348 patients who underwent preoperative lymphoscintigraphy and 240 patients who did not. The use of lymphoscintigraphy was not associated with a statistically significant advantage. Given this result and the sensitivity of intraoperative gamma probe identification of radioactive tracer uptake,[52] the role of preoperative lymphoscintigraphy has diminished at many centers. There is some evidence that patients who develop recurrent disease after breast-conserving therapy with axillary dissection or sentinel lymph node biopsy may particularly benefit from lymphoscintigraphy, as the pattern of lymphatic drainage is unpredictable in such patients. Lymphoscintigraphy identifies higher rates of nonaxillary lymphatic drainage in these patients and may guide therapy.[53]

Some centers have advocated 2-day protocols in which radioisotope is injected on the day before operation as opposed to the more common same-day approach. Such an approach potentially obviates the occasional delays associated with same-day injection and lymphoscintigraphy. Potential disadvantages of a 2-day protocol include a requirement for higher doses of radioisotope; passage of radioisotope into higher-echelon nodes, making identification of sentinel nodes more challenging; and inconvenience for patients. The feasibility and reliability of a 2-day protocol has been confirmed in several studies.[54–56] In one study, by McCarter and colleagues,[55] 1-day and 2-day protocols were compared: 933 patients received technetium-99 the day of operation and 387 patients received technetium-99 the day before operation. The mean number of sentinel lymph nodes identified was slightly higher in the former group.

IMMEDIATE PATHOLOGIC ASSESSMENT OF THE SENTINEL NODE

The benefit of an immediate pathologic assessment of a sentinel node remains somewhat controversial. The advantage of such an assessment is obvious; it allows for immediate completion axillary dissection if a sentinel node biopsy is positive, sparing the patient a second operation. False-positive results, however, may lead to unnecessary operations with associated morbidity. Studies of frozen sections in this setting do not justify the latter concern; a sensitivity of 76% and specificity of 99% are reported.[57] Moreover, rapid immunohistochemistry, serial sectioning, and real-time polymerase chain reaction assays may increase the accuracy of intraoperative pathologic assessment further. Despite this, there remains considerable variability in institutions regarding the use of immediate pathologic assessment.

CURRENT CONTROVERSIES
The Timing of Sentinel Lymph Node Biopsy in Patients Receiving Neoadjuvant Therapy

Neoadjuvant chemotherapy is increasingly used in the treatment of breast cancers. Moreover, the indications for this approach have expanded to include patients with less advanced disease. For these reasons, more patients with clinically node-positive and node-negative disease receive preoperative chemotherapy, many of whom require axillary staging. The optimal timing of sentinel lymph node biopsy in such patients is a subject of active debate. Sentinel lymph node biopsy before administration of neoadjuvant therapy may allow accurate nodal assessment before the lymphatics are compromised by the effects of chemotherapy. This accurate staging may simplify surgical management after chemotherapy; patients with a negative sentinel node biopsy can forgo axillary dissection. It also has been argued that nodal staging before chemotherapy provides important prognostic information and may predict the risk of treatment failure.[58]

Alternatively, axillary staging after chemotherapy may better reflect downstaged disease, allowing less aggressive surgical management.

Rates of sentinel node identification before or after chemotherapy have been compared. Jones and colleagues reported a significantly better rate of identification when mapping was performed before chemotherapy (100% versus 81%). The false-negative rate in patients who were successfully mapped after chemotherapy was 11%. In patients with clinically node-positive disease before neoadjuvant therapy, rates of sentinel node identification after chemotherapy ranged from 69% to 100% with false-negative rates from 0% to 30%.[59] Recently, Le Bouedec and colleagues[60] identified an association between false-negative results and larger tumor size or clinical positive nodal status before chemotherapy. No consensus exists regarding the optimal timing of axillary staging in patients receiving neoadjuvant chemotherapy; however, these data suggest that clinicians can anticipate a higher rate of false-negative results associated with sentinel lymph node biopsy after chemotherapy. The American College of Surgeons Oncology Group (ACOSOG) is currently conducting a study, Z1071, that specifically evaluates the accuracy of sentinel lymph node biopsy in patients with node-positive breast cancer after neoadjuvant therapy. In the near future there will be data that define sentinel node identification rates and accuracy after neoadjuvant chemotherapy.

The Need for Completion Dissection after a Positive Sentinel Lymph Node Biopsy

Completion axillary dissection remains the standard of care in those cases in which a sentinel lymph node biopsy contains metastases. More recently, this practice has been called into question. As many as 50% of patients with sentinel nodes containing metastases have no other axillary metastases.[61] Moreover, the absolute impact of axillary dissection on disease-free and overall survival has not been definitively quantified. Some observational studies have suggested low rates of local recurrence or distant metastases in patients with sentinel node metastases who declined or could not undergo completion dissection.[62] A meta-analysis examining whether or not prophylactic axillary dissection confers any survival advantage for patients with invasive breast cancer suggested a survival advantage of approximately 5% in the group of patients that underwent axillary dissection. Fewer patients included in the analysis, however, received adjuvant therapy than would have today. This issue

Table 1
Fluorine-18 fluorodeoxyglucose–positron emission tomography scanning in detection of sentinel lymph node and axillary lymph node metastasis in breast cancer patients

Author	Year	Number of Patients	Sensitivity (%)	Specificity (%)
Adler et al[107]	1993	20	90	100
Crowe et al[76]	1994	20	90	100
Avril et al[77]	1996	41	79	100
Scheidhauer et al[78]	1996	18	100	89
Utech et al[79]	1996	124	100	75
Crippa et al[80]	1997	82	84	85
Adler et al[81]	1997	50	95	66
Crippa et al[82]	1998	72	85	91
Noh et al[83]	1998	27	93	100
Smith et al[84]	1998	50	90	97
Yutani et al[85]	2000	38	50	100
Greco et al[12]	2001	167	94	86
Schirrmeister et al[86]	2001	117	79	93
Yang et al[87]	2001	18	50	100
Guller et al[88]	2002	31	43	94
Kelemen et al[89]	2002	15	20	90
van der Hoeven et al[90]	2002	70	25	97
Barranger et al[91]	2003	32	20	100
Wahl et al[92]	2004	360	61	80
Fehr et al[93]	2004	24	20	93
Zornoza et al[94]	2004	200	84	98
Lovrics et al[95]	2004	98	40	97
Chung et al[96]	2006	51	60	100
Kumar et al[97]	2006	80	44	95
Stadnik et al[98]	2006	10	80	100
Gil-Rendo et al[99]	2006	275	84	98
Veronesi et al[100]	2007	236	37	96
Mustafa et al[101]	2007	27	83	100
Ueda et al[102]	2008	183	58	95
Taira et al[103]	2009	92	48	92
Kim et al[104]	2009	137	77	100
Chae et al[105]	2009	108	48	84
Heusner et al[106]	2009	61	58	92

has been further complicated by the early closing of the ACOSOG-Z0011 trial due to slow patient accrual and a low number of events. This trial randomized patients with T1 or T2 tumors treated with breast-conserving therapy with clinically negative axillae and a single sentinel lymph node metastases to completion axillary dissection and adjuvant therapy or adjuvant therapy alone.[63] In the absence of higher-level evidence, this issue will likely remain unresolved.

Micrometastases

Adding further to the controversy over the indications for completion axillary dissection in patients with sentinel lymph node metastases is the increased identification of small foci of metastatic disease. These foci are characterized as micrometastases when they are less than or equal to 2 mm in diameter or submicrometastases when[64] less than or equal to 0.2 mm in diameter. This issue is

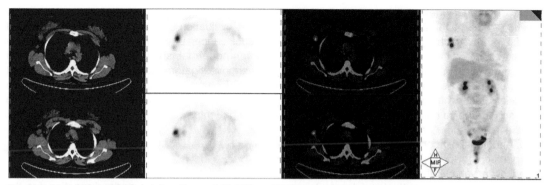

Fig. 1. True positive PET/CT. Axial sections of CT, PET, and PET/CT showing nodule in upper outer quadrant of right breast on CT; FDG uptake was noted on PET and PET/CT images in the nodule (*upper row*). Right axillary node seen on CT image shows FDG uptake in PET and PET/CT images (*lower row*). Projection image shows increased FDG uptake in primary breast cancer and metastatic axillary lymph node.

complicated by the limitations of pathologic assessment of the axillary contents (less exhaustive than the assessment of the sentinel node), which limits the accuracy of data on the presence of additional metastatic disease in patients undergoing completion dissection after a positive sentinel lymph node biopsy. The retrospective data on this subject remain contradictory. Several investigators have questioned the utility of completion dissection, particularly in patients with submillimeter metastases.[65] Conversely, Veronesi and colleagues[66] reported a 17% incidence of additional nodal metastases in patients with micrometastases in the sentinel node. Although

ongoing randomized trials (eg, the ACOSOG-Z0010 trial) may yield more definitive answers on this subject,[67] most institutions advocate completion dissection for patients with micrometastatic disease in a sentinel lymph node.

Predicting the Presence of Nonsentinel Nodal Metastases

A trend toward the more selective application of regional lymphadenectomy has prompted investigators to identify factors associated with a lower likelihood of nonsentinel nodal metastases in patients with a positive sentinel lymph node

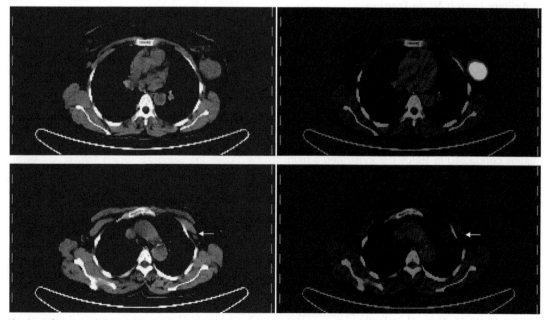

Fig. 2. False-negative PET/CT. Axial section of CT and PET/CT images showing nodule in upper outer quadrant of left breast with FDG uptake on PET/CT image (*upper row*). Small subcentimeter left axillary node seen on CT (*arrow*) does not take up FDG on PET/CT (*lower row*). The sentinel lymph node biopsy revealed a metastasis.

biopsy. These include small tumor size and the absence of sentinel node metastases greater than 2.0 mm.[68] Recently, several tools have been designed to allow the prediction of nonsentinel nodal metastases in patients with positive sentinel nodes, including several nomograms (eg, the Memorial Sloan-Kettering Cancer Center nomogram and the Mayo nomogram), scoring systems (eg, the Tenon score and the University of Texas M. D. Anderson Cancer Center score), and recursive partitioning tools. These tools calculate risk based on a variety of parameters, including, in some cases, number of sentinel nodal metastases, size of the metastases, presence of lymphovascular invasion, and size of the primary tumor. The Memorial Sloan-Kettering Cancer Center nomogram was studied by Alran and colleagues,[69] who suggested that it was more reliable for patients with macrometastasis than macrometastasis. Subsequently, a prospective multicenter study compared nine predictive tools. The investigators showed that the Tenon score is particularly accurate in identifying patients with micrometastasis and a low probability of additional metastases. The Memorial Sloan-Kettering Cancer Center and Stanford nomograms also performed well in this regard, in contradiction to the Alran and colleagues study.[70–75]

The Role of Positron Emission Tomography and Positron Emission Tomography/CT in Axillary Lymph Node Staging

Recently, PET has emerged as an important diagnostic imaging modality in the management of various cancers. Although PET alone is limited in its ability to localize focal areas of fluorine-18 fluorodeoxyglucose (FDG) uptake, the addition of CT to PET imaging (PET/CT) allows for more accurate localization. Many investigators have studied the role of PET using FDG in the management of patients with breast cancer (**Table 1**).[12,76–106] Studies conducted in 1990s demonstrated a high sensitivity and specificity of FDG-PET in assessing the status of axillary lymph nodes (**Fig. 1**).[76–84,107] More recent studies comparing the accuracy of FDG-PET to that of sentinel lymph node biopsy or axillary node dissection have yielded conflicting results (**Fig. 2**).[12,85–106] These divergent findings may reflect, in part, the use of immunohistochemical analysis and multistep sectioning of sentinel nodes in some studies, which detect micrometastasis and upstage disease in up to 46% of patients.[75,108,109] The role of sentinel lymph node biopsy for staging the axilla in breast cancer has now been well established; FDG-PET or PET/CT cannot replace

histologic staging but may play an important role in the evaluation of patients with locally advanced breast cancer in whom the incidence of axillary lymph node metastases is high. The authors and other investigators demonstrated that PET and PET/CT have a high-specificity and positive predictive value when used to stage the axilla in such patients.[95–101]

SUMMARY

Sentinel lymph node biopsy has largely supplanted elective lymph node dissection for the staging of invasive breast cancer. This procedure has been validated through multiple randomized trials and allows accurate prediction of the presence of axillary metastases. Although the procedure has been refined over the past decade, several technical aspects, including the optimal site of, timing of, and agents used for injection remain controversial. Similarly, the indications for sentinel lymph node biopsy in patients with early disease and implication of micrometastasis and submicrometastasis in the sentinel node remain areas of active investigation. The role of sentinel lymph node biopsy before and after neoadjuvant chemotherapy is currently being explored.

REFERENCES

1. Carter CL, Allen C, Henson DE. Relation of tumor size, lymph node status, and survival in 24,740 breast cancer cases. Cancer 1989;63:181–7.
2. Wilking N, Rutqvist LE, Carstensen J, et al. Prognostic significance of axillary nodal status in primary breast cancer in relation to the number of resected nodes. Stockholm Breast Cancer Study Group. Acta Oncol 1992;31:29–35.
3. Fisher B, Bauer M, Wickerham DL, et al. Relation of number of positive axillary nodes to the prognosis of patients with primary breast cancer. An NSABP update. Cancer 1983;52:1551–7.
4. Rosen PP, Saigo PE, Braun DW, et al. Axillary micro- and macrometastases in breast cancer: prognostic significance of tumor size. Ann Surg 1981;194:585–91.
5. Huvos AG, Hutter RV, Berg JW. Significance of axillary macrometastases and micrometastases in mammary cancer. Ann Surg 1971;173:44–6.
6. Donegan WL, Stine SB, Samter TG. Implications of extracapsular nodal metastases for treatment and prognosis of breast cancer. Cancer 1993;72:778–82.
7. Chadha M, Chabon AB, Friedmann P, et al. Predictors of axillary lymph node metastases in patients with T1 breast cancer. A multivariate analysis. Cancer 1994;73:350–3.

8. Menard S, Bufalino R, Rilke F, et al. Prognosis based on primary breast carcinoma instead of pathological nodal status. Br J Cancer 1994;70: 709–12.

9. Ravdin PM, De Laurentiis M, Vendely T, et al. Prediction of axillary lymph node status in breast cancer patients by use of prognostic indicators. J Natl Cancer Inst 1994;86:1771–5.

10. Allan SM. The prospects for imaging lymph nodes in breast cancer. Eur J Nucl Med 1992;19:836–7.

11. Nieweg OE, Kim EE, Wong WH, et al. Positron emission tomography with fluorine-18-deoxyglucose in the detection and staging of breast cancer. Cancer 1993;71:3920–5.

12. Greco M, Crippa F, Agresti R, et al. Axillary lymph node staging in breast cancer by 2-fluoro-2-deoxy-D-glucose-positron emission tomography: clinical evaluation and alternative management. J Natl Cancer Inst 2001;93:630–5.

13. Mameri CS, Kemp C, Goldman SM, et al. Impact of breast MRI on surgical treatment, axillary approach, and systemic therapy for breast cancer. Breast J 2008;14:236–44.

14. Cabanas RM. An approach for the treatment of penile carcinoma. Cancer 1977;39:456–66.

15. Morton DL, Wen DR, Foshag LJ, et al. Intraoperative lymphatic mapping and selective cervical lymphadenectomy for early-stage melanomas of the head and neck. J Clin Oncol 1993;11:1751–6.

16. Morton DL, Thompson JF, Essner R, et al. Validation of the accuracy of intraoperative lymphatic mapping and sentinel lymphadenectomy for early-stage melanoma: a multicenter trial. Multicenter Selective Lymphadenectomy Trial Group. Ann Surg 1999;230:453–63 [discussion: 63–5].

17. Giuliano AE, Jones RC, Brennan M, et al. Sentinel lymphadenectomy in breast cancer. J Clin Oncol 1997;15:2345–50.

18. Krag D, Weaver D, Ashikaga T, et al. The sentinel node in breast cancer—a multicenter validation study. N Engl J Med 1998;339:941–6.

19. Veronesi U, Paganelli G, Viale G, et al. Sentinel lymph node biopsy and axillary dissection in breast cancer: results in a large series. J Natl Cancer Inst 1999;91:368–73.

20. Green M, Farshid G, Kollias J, et al. The tissue distribution of Evans blue dye in a sheep model of sentinel node biopsy. Nucl Med Commun 2006; 27:695–700.

21. Faries MB, Bedrosian I, Reynolds C, et al. Active macromolecule uptake by lymph node antigen-presenting cells: a novel mechanism in determining sentinel lymph node status. Ann Surg Oncol 2000;7:98–105.

22. Barth A, Craig PH, Silverstein MJ. Predictors of axillary lymph node metastases in patients with T1 breast carcinoma. Cancer 1997;79:1918–22.

23. Voogd AC, Coebergh JW, Repelaer van Driel OJ, et al. The risk of nodal metastases in breast cancer patients with clinically negative lymph nodes: a population-based analysis. Breast Cancer Res Treat 2000;62:63–9.

24. Javid SH, Smith BL, Mayer E, et al. Tubular carcinoma of the breast: results of a large contemporary series. Am J Surg 2009;197:674–7.

25. Huo L, Sneige N, Hunt KK, et al. Predictors of invasion in patients with core-needle biopsy-diagnosed ductal carcinoma in situ and recommendations for a selective approach to sentinel lymph node biopsy in ductal carcinoma in situ. Cancer 2006;107: 1760–8.

26. Yen TW, Hunt KK, Ross MI, et al. Predictors of invasive breast cancer in patients with an initial diagnosis of ductal carcinoma in situ: a guide to selective use of sentinel lymph node biopsy in management of ductal carcinoma in situ. J Am Coll Surg 2005;200:516–26.

27. Roses RE, Paulson EC, Sharma A, et al. HER-2/neu overexpression as a predictor for the transition from in situ to invasive breast cancer. Cancer Epidemiol Biomarkers Prev 2009;18:1386–9.

28. Liu LC, Lang JE, Jenkins T, et al. Is it necessary to harvest additional lymph nodes after resection of the most radioactive sentinel lymph node in breast cancer? J Am Coll Surg 2008;207:853–8.

29. Kesmodel SB, Canter RJ, Terhune KP, et al. Use of radiotracer for sentinel lymph node mapping in breast cancer optimizes staging independent of site of administration. Clin Nucl Med 2006;31: 527–33.

30. Krag DN, Weaver DL, Alex JC, et al. Surgical resection and radiolocalization of the sentinel lymph node in breast cancer using a gamma probe. Surg Oncol 1993;2:335–9 [discussion: 40].

31. Linehan DC, Hill AD, Tran KN, et al. Sentinel lymph node biopsy in breast cancer: unfiltered radioisotope is superior to filtered. J Am Coll Surg 1999; 188:377–81.

32. Mariani G, Erba P, Villa G, et al. Lymphoscintigraphic and intraoperative detection of the sentinel lymph node in breast cancer patients: the nuclear medicine perspective. J Surg Oncol 2004;85: 112–22.

33. Ellner SJ, Hoh CK, Vera DR, et al. Dose-dependent biodistribution of [(99m)Tc]DTPA-mannosyl-dextran for breast cancer sentinel lymph node mapping. Nucl Med Biol 2003;30:805–10.

34. Wallace AM, Hoh CK, Ellner SJ, et al. Lymphoseek: a molecular imaging agent for melanoma sentinel lymph node mapping. Ann Surg Oncol 2007;14: 913–21.

35. Takagi K, Uehara T, Kaneko E, et al. 99mTc-labeled mannosyl-neoglycoalbumin for sentinel lymph

node identification. Nucl Med Biol 2004;31: 893–900.

36. Jeong JM, Hong MK, Kim YJ, et al. Development of 99mTc-neomannosyl human serum albumin (99mTc-MSA) as a novel receptor binding agent for sentinel lymph node imaging. Nucl Med Commun 2004;25:1211–7.

37. Giuliano AE, Kirgan DM, Guenther JM, et al. Lymphatic mapping and sentinel lymphadenectomy for breast cancer. Ann Surg 1994;220:391–8 [discussion: 8–401].

38. Raut CP, Hunt KK, Akins JS, et al. Incidence of anaphylactoid reactions to isosulfan blue dye during breast carcinoma lymphatic mapping in patients treated with preoperative prophylaxis: results of a surgical prospective clinical practice protocol. Cancer 2005;104:692–9.

39. Kuerer HM, Wayne JD, Ross MI. Anaphylaxis during breast cancer lymphatic mapping. Surgery 2001;129:119–20.

40. Blessing WD, Stolier AJ, Teng SC, et al. A comparison of methylene blue and lymphazurin in breast cancer sentinel node mapping. Am J Surg 2002; 184:341–5.

41. Chagpar A, Martin RC 3rd, Chao C, et al. Validation of subareolar and periareolar injection techniques for breast sentinel lymph node biopsy. Arch Surg 2004;139:614–8 [discussion: 8–20].

42. Chagpar AB, Martin RC, Scoggins CR, et al. Factors predicting failure to identify a sentinel lymph node in breast cancer. Surgery 2005;138: 56–63.

43. Borgstein PJ, Meijer S, Pijpers R. Intradermal blue dye to identify sentinel lymph-node in breast cancer. Lancet 1997;349:1668–9.

44. Martin RC, Derossis AM, Fey J, et al. Intradermal isotope injection is superior to intramammary in sentinel node biopsy for breast cancer. Surgery 2001;130:432–8.

45. Bauer TW, Spitz FR, Callans LS, et al. Subareolar and peritumoral injection identify similar sentinel nodes for breast cancer. Ann Surg Oncol 2002;9: 169–76.

46. Klimberg VS, Rubio IT, Henry R, et al. Subareolar versus peritumoral injection for location of the sentinel lymph node. Ann Surg 1999;229:860–4 [discussion: 4–5].

47. Newman EA, Newman LA. Lymphatic mapping techniques and sentinel lymph node biopsy in breast cancer. Surg Clin North Am 2007;87: 353–64, viii.

48. Jansen L, Doting MH, Rutgers EJ, et al. Clinical relevance of sentinel lymph nodes outside the axilla in patients with breast cancer. Br J Surg 2000;87: 920–5.

49. Klauber-DeMore N, Bevilacqua JL, Van Zee KJ, et al. Comprehensive review of the management of internal mammary lymph node metastases in breast cancer. J Am Coll Surg 2001;193:547–55.

50. Noguchi M. Relevance and practicability of internal mammary sentinel node biopsy for breast cancer. Breast Cancer 2002;9:329–36.

51. McMasters KM, Wong SL, Tuttle TM, et al. Preoperative lymphoscintigraphy for breast cancer does not improve the ability to identify axillary sentinel lymph nodes. Ann Surg 2000;231:724–31.

52. Borgstein PJ, Pijpers R, Comans EF, et al. Sentinel lymph node biopsy in breast cancer: guidelines and pitfalls of lymphoscintigraphy and gamma probe detection. J Am Coll Surg 1998;186:275–83.

53. Port ER, Garcia-Etienne CA, Park J, et al. Reoperative sentinel lymph node biopsy: a new frontier in the management of ipsilateral breast tumor recurrence. Ann Surg Oncol 2007;14:2209–14.

54. Winchester DJ, Sener SF, Winchester DP, et al. Sentinel lymphadenectomy for breast cancer: experience with 180 consecutive patients: efficacy of filtered technetium 99m sulphur colloid with overnight migration time. J Am Coll Surg 1999;188:597–603.

55. McCarter MD, Yeung H, Yeh S, et al. Localization of the sentinel node in breast cancer: identical results with same-day and day-before isotope injection. Ann Surg Oncol 2001;8:682–6.

56. Solorzano CC, Ross MI, Delpassand E, et al. Utility of breast sentinel lymph node biopsy using day-before-surgery injection of high-dose 99mTc-labeled sulfur colloid. Ann Surg Oncol 2001;8:821–7.

57. Viale G, Bosari S, Mazzarol G, et al. Intraoperative examination of axillary sentinel lymph nodes in breast carcinoma patients. Cancer 1999;85: 2433–8.

58. Kilbride KE, Lee MC, Nees AV, et al. Axillary staging prior to neoadjuvant chemotherapy for breast cancer: predictors of recurrence. Ann Surg Oncol 2008;15:3252–8.

59. Straver ME, Rutgers EJ, Russell NS, et al. Towards rational axillary treatment in relation to neoadjuvant therapy in breast cancer. Eur J Cancer 2009.

60. Le Bouedec G, Geissler B, Gimbergues P, et al. Sentinel lymph node biopsy for breast cancer after neoadjuvant chemotherapy: influence of nodal status before treatment. Bull Cancer 2006;93: 415–9.

61. Goyal A, Douglas-Jones A, Newcombe RG, et al. Predictors of non-sentinel lymph node metastasis in breast cancer patients. Eur J Cancer 2004;40: 1731–7.

62. Guenther JM, Hansen NM, DiFronzo LA, et al. Axillary dissection is not required for all patients with breast cancer and positive sentinel nodes. Arch Surg 2003;138:52–6.

63. Ross MI. Sentinel node dissection in early-stage breast cancer: ongoing prospective randomized trials in the USA. Ann Surg Oncol 2001;8:77S–81S.

64. Jones JL, Zabicki K, Christian RL, et al. A comparison of sentinel node biopsy before and after neoadjuvant chemotherapy: timing is important. Am J Surg 2005;190:517–20.

65. Fournier K, Schiller A, Perry RR, et al. Micrometastasis in the sentinel lymph node of breast cancer does not mandate completion axillary dissection. Ann Surg 2004;239:859–63 [discussion: 63–5].

66. Veronesi U, Paganelli G, Viale G, et al. A randomized comparison of sentinel-node biopsy with routine axillary dissection in breast cancer. N Engl J Med 2003;349:546–53.

67. White RL Jr, Wilke LG. Update on the NSABP and ACOSOG breast cancer sentinel node trials. Am J Surg 2004;70:420–4.

68. Reynolds C, Mick R, Donohue JH, et al. Sentinel lymph node biopsy with metastasis: can axillary dissection be avoided in some patients with breast cancer? J Clin Oncol 1999;17:1720–6.

69. Alran S, De Rycke Y, Fourchotte V, et al. Validation and limitations of use of a breast cancer nomogram predicting the likelihood of non-sentinel node involvement after positive sentinel node biopsy. Ann Surg Oncol 2007;14:2195–201.

70. Coutant C, Olivier C, Lambaudie E, et al. Comparison of models to predict nonsentinel lymph node status in breast cancer patients with metastatic sentinel lymph nodes: a prospective multicenter study. J Clin Oncol 2009;27:2800–8.

71. Krak NC, van der Hoeven JJ, Hoekstra OS, et al. Measuring [(18)F]FDG uptake in breast cancer during chemotherapy: comparison of analytical methods. Eur J Nucl Med Mol Imaging 2003;30:674–81.

72. Kao CH, Hsieh JF, Tsai SC, et al. Comparison and discrepancy of 18F-2-deoxyglucose positron emission tomography and Tc-99m MDP bone scan to detect bone metastasis. Anticancer Res 2000;20:2189–92.

73. Kostakoglu L, Goldsmith SJ. 18F-FDG PET evaluation of the response to therapy for lymphoma and for breast, lung, and colorectal carcinoma. J Nucl Med 2003;44:224–39.

74. Eubank WB, Mankoff DA, Vesselle HJ, et al. Detection of locoregional and distant recurrences in breast cancer patients by using FDG PET. Radiographics 2002;22:5–17.

75. Dowlatshahi K, Fan M, Bloom K, et al. Occult metastasis in the sentinel lymph nodes of patients with early stage breast carcinoma. A preliminary study. Cancer 1999;86:990–6.

76. Crowe JP Jr, Adler LP, Shenk RR, et al. Positron emission tomography and breast masses: comparison with clinical, mammographic, and pathological findings. Ann Surg Oncol 1994;1:132–40.

77. Avril N, Dose J, Janicke F, et al. Assessment of axillary lymph node involvement in breast cancer patients with positron emission tomography using radiolabeled 2-(fluorine-18)-fluoro-2-deoxy-D-glucose. J Natl Cancer Inst 1996;88:1204–9.

78. Scheidhauer K, Scharl A, Pietrzyk U, et al. Qualitative [18F]FDG positron emission tomography in primary breast cancer: clinical relevance and practicability. Eur J Nucl Med 1996;23:618–23.

79. Utech CI, Young CS, Winter PF. Prospective evaluation of fluorine-18 fluorodeoxyclucose positron emission tomography in breast cancer for staging of the axilla related to surgery and immunocytochemistry. Eur J Nucl Med 1996;23:1588–93.

80. Crippa F, Agresti R, Donne VD, et al. The contribution of positron emission tomography (PET) with 18F-fluorodeoxyglucose (FDG) in the preoperative detection of axillary metastasis of breast cancer: the experience of the National Cancer Institute of Milan. Tumori 1997;83:542–3.

81. Adler LP, Faulhaber PF, Schnur KC, et al. Axillary lymph node metastasis: screening with [F-18]2-deoxy-2-fluoro-D-glucose (FDG) PET. Radiology 1997;203:323–7.

82. Crippa F, Agresti R, Seregni E, et al. Prospective evaluation of fluorine-18-FDG PET in presurgical staging of the axilla in breast cancer. J Nucl Med 1998;39:4–8.

83. Noh DY, Yun IJ, Kim JS, et al. Diagnostic value of positron emission tomography for detecting breast cancer. World J Surg 1998;22:223–7.

84. Smith IC, Ogston KN, Whitford P, et al. Staging of the axilla in breast cancer: accurate in vivo assessment using positron emission tomography with 2-(fluorine-18)-fluoro-2-deoxy-D-glucose. Ann Surg 1998;228:220–7.

85. Yutani K, Shiba E, Kusuoka H, et al. Comparison of FDG–PET with MIBI-SPECT in the detection of breast cancer and axillary lymph node metastasis. J Comput Assist Tomogr 2000;24:274–80.

86. Schirrmeister H, Kuhn T, Guhlmann A, et al. Fluorine-18 2-deoxy-2-fluoro-D-glucose PET in the preoperative staging of breast cancer: comparison with the standard staging procedures. Eur J Nucl Med 2001;28:351–8.

87. Yang JH, Nam SJ, Lee TS, et al. Comparison of intraoperative frozen section analysis of sentinel node with preoperative positron emission tomography in the diagnosis of axillary lymph node status in breast cancer patients. Jpn J Clin Oncol 2001;31:1–6.

88. Guller U, Nitzsche EU, Schirp U, et al. Selective axillary surgery in breast cancer patients based on positron emission tomography with 18F-fluoro-2-deoxy-D-glucose: not yet!. Breast Cancer Res Treat 2002;71:171–3.

89. Kelemen PR, Lowe V, Phillips N. Positron emission tomography and sentinel lymph node

dissection in breast cancer. Clin Breast Cancer 2002;3:73–7.

90. van der Hoeven JJ, Hoekstra OS, Comans EF, et al. Determinants of diagnostic performance of [F-18]fluorodeoxyglucose positron emission tomography for axillary staging in breast cancer. Ann Surg 2002;236:619–24.

91. Barranger E, Grahek D, Antoine M, et al. Evaluation of fluorodeoxyglucose positron emission tomography in the detection of axillary lymph node metastasis in patients with early-stage breast cancer. Ann Surg Oncol 2003;10:622–7.

92. Wahl RL, Siegel BA, Coleman RE, et al. PET Study Group. Prospective multicenter study of axillary nodal staging by positron emission tomography in breast cancer: a report of the staging breast cancer with PET Study Group. J Clin Oncol 2004; 22:277–85.

93. Fehr MK, Hornung R, Varga Z, et al. Axillary staging using positron emission tomography in breast cancer patients qualifying for sentinel lymph node biopsy. Breast J 2004;10:89–93.

94. Zornoza G, Garcia-Velloso MJ, Sola J, et al. 18F-FDG PET complemented with sentinel lymph node biopsy in the detection of axillary involvement in breast cancer. Eur J Surg Oncol 2004;30:15–9.

95. Lovrics PJ, Chen V, Coates G, et al. A prospective evaluation of positron emission tomography scanning, sentinel lymph node biopsy, and standard axillary dissection for axillary staging in patients with early stage breast cancer. Ann Surg Oncol 2004;11:846–53.

96. Chung A, Liou D, Karlan S, et al. Preoperative FDG-PET for axillary metastases in patients with breast cancer. Arch Surg 2006;141(8):783–8.

97. Kumar R, Zhuang H, Schnall M, et al. Alavi A.FDG PET positive lymph nodes are highly predictive of metastasis in breast cancer. Nucl Med Commun 2006;27(3):231–6.

98. Stadnik TW, Everaert H, Makkat S, et al. Breast imaging. Preoperative breast cancer staging: comparison of USPIO-enhanced MR imaging and 18F-fluorodeoxyglucose (FDC) positron emission tomography (PET) imaging for axillary lymph node staging–initial findings. Eur Radiol 2006; 16(10):2153–60.

99. Gil-Rendo A, Zornoza G, García-Velloso MJ, et al. Fluorodeoxyglucose positron emission tomography with sentinel lymph node biopsy for evaluation of axillary involvement in breast cancer. Br J Surg 2006;93(6):707–12.

100. Veronesi U, De Cicco C, Galimberti VE, et al. A comparative study on the value of FDG-PET and sentinel node biopsy to identify occult axillary metastases. Ann Oncol 2007;18(3):473–8.

101. Mustafa S, Marshall C, Griffiths PA, et al. Eremin O.18F-FDG dual-headed gamma camera PET in detection of axillary nodal disease in patients with large or locally advanced breast cancer: possible alternative staging of axilla. Oncol Rep 2007;18(6):1545–9.

102. Ueda S, Tsuda H, Asakawa H, et al. Utility of 18F-fluoro-deoxyglucose emission tomography/ computed tomography fusion imaging (18F-FDG PET/CT) in combination with ultrasonography for axillary staging in primary breast cancer. BMC Cancer 2008;8:165.

103. Taira N, Ohsumi S, Takabatake D, et al. Determination of indication for sentinel lymph node biopsy in clinical node-negative breast cancer using preoperative 18F-fluorodeoxyglucose positron emission tomography/computed tomography fusion imaging. Jpn J Clin Oncol 2009;39(1): 16–21.

104. Kim J, Lee J, Chang E, et al. Selective sentinel node plus additional non-sentinel node biopsy based on an FDG-PET/CT scan in early breast cancer patients: single institutional experience. World J Surg 2009;33(5):943–9.

105. Chae BJ, Bae JS, Kang BJ, et al. Jpn Positron emission tomography-computed tomography in the detection of axillary lymph node metastasis in patients with early stage breast cancer. J Clin Oncol 2009;39(5):284–9.

106. Heusner TA, Kuemmel S, Umutlu L, et al. Breast cancer staging in a single session: whole-body PET/CT mammography. J Nucl Med 2008;49(8): 1215–22.

107. Adler LP, Crowe JP, al-Kaisi NK, et al. Evaluation of breast masses and axillary lymph nodes with [F-18] 2-deoxy-2-fluoro-D-glucose PET. Radiology 1993;187:743–50.

108. Turner RR, Chu KU, Qi K, et al. Pathologic features associated with nonsentinel lymph node metastasis in patients with metastatic breast carcinoma in a sentinel lymph node. Cancer 2000;89:574–81.

109. Freneaux P, Nos C, Vincent-Salomon A, et al. Histological detection of minimal metastatic involvement in axillary sentinel nodes: a rational basis for a sensitive methodology usable in daily practice. Mod Pathol 2002;15:641–6.

The Role of PET and PET/CT in the Surgical Management of Breast Cancer: A Review

Susan Bahl, MD[a],
Abass Alavi, MD, MD (Hon), PhD (Hon), DSc (Hon)[b],
Sandip Basu, MD[c], Rakesh Kumar, MD[d],
Brian J. Czerniecki, MD, PhD[a,e,*]

KEYWORDS

- PET • PET/CT • Breast cancer • Surgical management

Various imaging modalities are used in the diagnosis and treatment planning of the breast cancer patient. Mammography, breast ultrasound, and magnetic resonance imaging (MR imaging) are the primary diagnostic modalities to evaluate breast pathology. Although mammography remains the primary imaging modality used in the detection of early breast cancer, the incidence of false-negative results is estimated to be 5% to 15%.[1] The inability to detect breast cancer with mammography is multifactorial, often because of the superimposed fibroglandular tissue. This imperfect sensitivity of mammography has led to the use of use of adjunctive imaging methods, including MR imaging. Although MR imaging has demonstrated variable specificity, the reported sensitivity of this modality for the demonstration of invasive breast cancer has approached 100% in several series.[1]

^{18}F-FDG positron emission tomography (PET) and more recently, ^{18}F-FDG positron emission tomography/computed tomography (PET/CT) have now emerged as another imaging tool for many malignant neoplasms, including breast cancer. Malignant cells generally have enhanced glucose metabolism compared with nonmalignant cells, and therefore exhibit increased glycolytic activity. Malignant cells have substantially enhanced glucose transporters (GLUT) on their surface (mainly the GLUT 1 and GLUT 3 receptors). Malignant cells also express high levels of hexokinase and low levels of glucose-6-phosphatase, which lead to an enhanced glucose uptake of glucose in these cells. FDG is metabolized similar to that of glucose and as FDG enters the cell via glucose transporter proteins, it competes with glucose for hexokinase (which is overexpressed in the malignant cells), and is phosphorylated subsequently. In contrast to glucose-6-phosphate, however, FDG-6-phosphate is metabolically trapped within the tumor cells in proportion to the glucose metabolic rate, and thus PET can detect its accumulation in these cells over time. Hence, the FDG uptake into the malignant cells is a consequence of a tumor cell's increased expression of glucose transport and glycolytic activity. As FDG accumulates, the contrast between lesions and the normal surrounding tissue increases. This leads to their prominent visualization of lesions on FDG-PET imaging. There is quite often substantial overlap between standardized uptake values (SUVs)

[a] The Department of Surgery, University of Pennsylvania School of Medicine, 34 West Spruce Street, Philadelphia, PA 19104, USA
[b] Department Section, Radiology, University of Pennsylvania School of Medicine, Philadelphia, PA, USA
[c] Radiation Medicine Centre, BARC, Mumbai, India
[d] Department of Nuclear Medicine, All India Institute of Medical Sciences, New Delhi-110029, India
[e] Department of Surgery, 3 Perelman Center, University of Pennsylvania School of Medicine, 3400 Civic Center Drive, Philadelphia, PA 19104, USA
* Corresponding author: Department of Surgery, 3 Perelman Center, 3400 Civic Center Drive, Philadelphia, PA 19104.
E-mail address: brian.czerniecki@uphs.upenn.edu (B.J. Czerniecki).

PET Clin 4 (2009) 277–287
doi:10.1016/j.cpet.2009.10.002

from active inflammatory processes (both of infectious and noninfectious origin) with those of malignant lesions. Therefore, a threshold value for SUV alone cannot be generally employed to differentiate between malignancy and benignity. However, inflammatory cells have higher levels of glucose-6-phosphatase than malignant cells, and therefore a lower ratio of hexokinase to glucose-6-phosphatase. Consequently, FDG-6-phosphate is rapidly dephosphorylated and cleared from the cell, leading to decreasing concentration of this metabolic product in these cells over time. In contrast, the most actively proliferating tumors tend to have the lowest levels of glucose-6-phosphatase. This difference forms the basis of dual time point FDG-PET in tumor cells.[2]

Minn and Soini[3] presented the first results obtained using FDG imaging in breast cancer in 1989. Most of the studies conducted since then have used 2-dimensional (2D) emission scanning, usually in conjunction with a separate transmission scan for attenuation correction. It is well known that attenuation correction is required for a quantitative assessment of tumor response to therapy and for accurate lesion localization.[2] Dual-modality PET/CT tomographs allow the simultaneous acquisition of anatomic and molecular information without moving the patient off and on the table in between examinations.[4] The CT transmission information can be used not only for anatomic localization and radiological assessment of lesions, but also for attenuation correction of the complementary emission data.

^{18}F-FDG PET has several advantages over other imaging modalities in cancer detection. Many forms of cancer are systemic and whole-body imaging with ^{18}F-FDG provides a noninvasive way to monitor extent and progression of the disease. Furthermore, because biochemical changes in a tumor occur in advance of morphologic changes, PET has the potential for greater sensitivity at an earlier stage of the disease.

The specificity of ^{18}F-FDG PET is limited because of the nonspecificity of FDG. FDG uptake in granulomatous disease, inflammation, post-therapeutic repair processes, muscles, and fat tissue may lead potentially to false positive results. With the introduction of PET/CT tomographs providing integrated anatomic and metabolic interpretation, false positive readings are expected to be reduced and the overall accuracy of diagnosis increased.

PET, PET/CT, AND DIAGNOSIS OF BREAST MALIGNANCY

Breast cancer often presents as a subcentimeter area of abnormality on screening mammography. An appropriate diagnostic modality must be able to demonstrate nonpalpable, small (<1.0 cm), invasive, and in situ malignancies. Most of the larger prospective studies using FDG-PET on patients with suspicious breast abnormalities by clinical or mammographic examinations have shown some of the limitations of FDG-PET in detecting (1) smaller (<1 cm) tumors, (2) more well-differentiated histologic subtypes of tumors (tubular carcinoma and in situ carcinoma), and (3) lobular carcinomas.[5] The overall sensitivities and specificities in these studies ranged from 80% to 100% and 75% to 100%, respectively.[6]

Diagnostic accuracy in PET appears to be dependent on tumor size. Many studies have analyzed the diagnostic accuracy of PET with relation to size of breast malignancy. Initial studies that included patients with advanced disease suggested high accuracy for the detection of primary breast carcinomas. For instance, Wahl and colleagues[7] correctly identified breast carcinomas in 10 patients with tumor sizes between 3 and 6 cm. Similarly, in a series of 28 patients, Adler and colleagues[8,9] found a sensitivity of 96% studying breast masses larger than 1 cm in diameter (**Fig. 1**). More recently in 2000, Avril and colleagues[6] investigated the value of PET in the diagnosis of breast carcinoma in 144 patients with suspicious masses on clinical examination. Images were analyzed for increased tracer uptake, applying conventional image-reading principles. Overall sensitivity was 65% to 80%, with a specificity of 76% to 94%

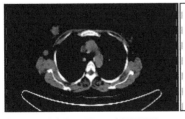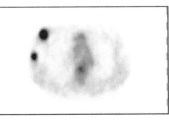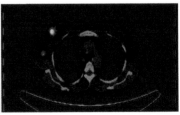

Fig. 1. Axial CT, PET, and PET/CT images of patient who presented with right breast nodule in upper outer quadrant. Focal area of intense FDG uptake was noted in primary breast cancer and right axially lymph node. Histopathology report was suggestive of primary ductal right breast cancer with right axillary lymph node metastasis.

depending on the visual assessment criteria used. The accuracy increased from 68% for T1 tumors to 92% for T2, and approached 100% for T3 tumors.[6] However, PET did not detect any of the four 0.5-cm tumors, and identified only one of eight tumors ranging from 0.5 to 1.0 cm. Although its overall sensitivity and specificity in detecting primary breast carcinoma appears to be acceptable, one must keep in mind that these data are mainly based on patients with large primary tumors. Therefore, the potential limitation of ^{18}F-FDG PET in diagnostic breast imaging is the detection of microscopic disease and lesions smaller than 1 cm (**Fig. 2**). As a result, ^{18}F-FDG PET is not routinely used in the staging work-up of patients with stage 1 or early stage 2 disease.

Variable metabolic activity intrinsic to each specific tumor type represents one of the most significant limitations for the routine diagnostic application of PET in breast carcinoma. These variations can lead to a wide array of SUV readings after administration of ^{18}F-FDG. To combat this issue, the technique of dual point imaging has been proposed. Most of the data involving the use of FDG-PET in breast carcinoma involves single time point imaging at 60 minutes after the administration of ^{18}F-FDG.[4] Dual point imaging involves measurement of uptake values at two separate time points following administration of FDG. Advantages of dual time point imaging have been demonstrated in head and neck, lung, pancreatic, and cervical malignancies. Similarly, it has been proposed that dual time point FDG-PET may improve the sensitivity and accuracy of FDG-PET in assessing patients with primary breast cancer.[10] In some tumors, the SUV does not reach maximum until 130 to 500 minutes after injection of ^{18}F-FDG. This is probably related to the increased glucose uptake through the glucose transporter proteins and low concentration of glucose-6-phosphatase activity in these cells.[4] In contrast, such a prolonged period of ^{18}F-FDG

uptake is rare in inflammatory lesions or normal tissues. The value obtained after the second time point can potentially heighten sensitivities of this imaging modality.

Various studies have demonstrated that the uptake of ^{18}F-FDG continues to rise in malignant tumors for several hours after the intravenous administration. In a 2006 study by Mavi and colleagues,[10] the authors were able to demonstrate that imaging at two different time points reveals substantially higher SUVs on delayed scans compared with those measured on the initial scans. The sensitivities of the dual time imaging method in detecting invasive cancer measuring larger than 10 mm, 4 to 10 mm, and noninvasive breast cancer were 90.1%, 82.7%, and 76.9%, respectively. In addition, invasive ductal cancer showed a significantly higher SUVmax1 value than those of invasive lobular and mixed types, which are relatively well-differentiated invasive cancers. Therefore, dual point imaging can result in higher SUV values, helping to differentiate between benign and malignant processes.

Recent technologic advances may improve primary breast tumor detection by PET. One prominent approach has been termed positron emission mammography (PEM). In this method, two planar detectors are integrated into a conventional mammographic system that enables co-registration of mammographic and emission FDG images of the breast.[11] The advantages of this dedicated system include improved geometric sensitivity, higher spatial resolution, shorter imaging time, and reduced attenuation compared with whole-body PET systems.[11] Although these dedicated breast-imaging systems have the potential capability to detect smaller and less FDG-avid breast tumors than conventional whole-body PET, their role in breast cancer screening or as a diagnostic adjunct to mammography is uncertain. It may be likely that certain early breast tumors are simply less glycolytic than larger lesions and will evade

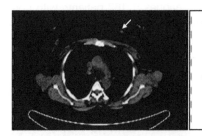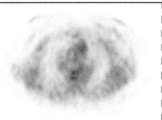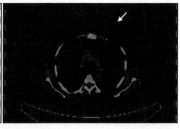

Fig. 2. Axial CT, PET, and PET/CT images of patient who presented with left breast nodule in inner quadrant. No FDG uptake was noted in the nodule (*arrow*) in PET/CT. Histopathology report was suggestive of primary ductal left breast cancer. PET/CT was false negative due to small tumor.

detection because of their inherent degree of FDG metabolism.

In summary, the ultimate role of FDG-PET in imaging primary breast lesions is not clear. It is not suited for screening purposes of primary breast cancer because of its high expense and modest whole-body radiation exposure. For diagnostic purposes in general screening, its accuracy does not appear comparable with the standard practice of mammography followed by targeted ultrasound examination. FDG-PET, particularly using the dual point method, may be helpful because of its high positive predictive value in selected patients. However, its role in primary tumor detection remains to be determined.

PET, PET/CT, AND AXILLARY NODAL STAGING

Axillary lymph node involvement is the most important prognostic factor in patients with breast cancer. Hence, accurate staging provides information to proceed with the correct surgical treatment plan. Because the extent of axillary disease influences the choice of therapeutic regimen for individual patients, a number of studies have evaluated the use of FDG-PET for axillary node staging. PET and PET/CT provide a whole body noninvasive technique to image for any loco regional or distant metastases. This single staging procedure theoretically offers an enormous advantage in the staging workup of the breast cancer patient.

Mammogram, ultrasound, and MR imaging do not allow for accurate evaluation of axillary lymph node status. At present, the technique of sentinel lymph node biopsy or formal axillary node dissection is used to determine the "N" stage. Sentinel lymph node biopsy (SLNB) is a selective sampling of the ipsilateral axillary lymph nodes deemed to primarily drain the lesion. These "sentinel" nodes are identified by using either or both a blue dye (lymphazurin blue or methylene blue) or a radionucleotide tracer (typically technetium sulfur colloid). In most series, using these mapping techniques, the accuracy of identifying the sentinel node approaches 95%.[12] This technique has the benefit of being a much less invasive procedure than a formal axillary dissection, with a lymphedema risk ranging from 2% to 5%; versus up to 25% for a standard axillary dissection.[12] In those patients in whom an SLNB cannot be performed, a standard axillary dissection is conducted. Both techniques provide detailed information regarding nodal histology. Nodes can be classified as either completely involving tumor, harboring a micro metastasis, or containing isolated tumor cells. This exquisite detail is available with the use of sensitive immunohistochemical staining of the nodal specimens.

PET and PET/CT can detect axillary involvement based on the hypermetabolic characteristics of the axillary nodal basins. Various studies have shown a relation between size of primary tumor and sensitivity of detection of axillary disease. In a study in 2004 by Lovrics and colleagues[13] a prospective evaluation of PET, SLN, and ALND was conducted in patients with early-stage breast cancer. This study compared preoperative FDG-PET with pathologic results from SLN biopsy in patients with early-stage breast cancer (**Fig. 3**). Sensitivities were found to be in the range of 20% to 50%. False negative FDG-PET results were seen predominantly in small-sized (10 mm or less) metastatic sentinel nodes.[13]

In another prospective study by Wahl and colleagues[14] that included a substantial proportion of patients with small primary tumors, FDG PET consistently underestimated the number of tumor-involved nodes compared with pathologic evaluation from conventional axillary dissection. Both of these studies showed that the sensitivity of FDG-PET in detecting axillary metastases is significantly less when only one node is positive versus several positive nodes and when the primary tumor has infiltrating lobular versus ductal histology.[14] These more recent studies demonstrate the limitation of PET's ability to detect small-volume axillary disease in early-stage breast cancer.

Patients with significant tumor burden within their axillary nodal basins may benefit from the use of PET/CT. In a recent prospective review by Cermik and colleagues,[15] 162 patients with core biopsy–proven breast malignancy were staged

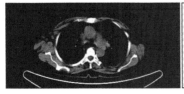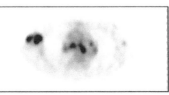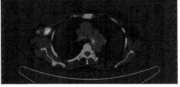

Fig. 3. Axial CT, PET, and PET/CT images of patient who presented with right breast cancer. FDG uptake was noted in multiple right axillary lymph nodes suggestive of metastatic lymphadenopathy.

using FDG-PET. The results revealed that FDG PET potentially upgraded TNM stage in 9.2% of patients. The sensitivity for detecting axillary lymph node metastasis was found to be 41% in pN1, 67% in pN2, and 100% in pN3, and the specificity was 89% for pN0 stage.[15] The data described indicate that FDG-PET imaging can detect axillary lymph node involvement with high sensitivity and specificity in patients with high axillary lymph node stages. However, detection rate of N1 axillary lymph node metastasis is low with current PET technology (see **Fig. 2**).

Although recent data do not support the routine use of FDG-PET for axillary staging of early breast cancer, FDG-PET may be complementary to SLN mapping and other standard axillary procedures in patients with more advanced tumors and/or equivocally palpable axillary nodes. Typically in advanced disease, an SLNB may be replaced by a large volume of disease and may not be visualized at mapping because lymph flow is diverted around it, resulting in a potential false negative examination. A clearly positive FDG-PET in selected patients with a high risk of nodal metastases carries high positive predictive value and may identify patients with evidence of nodal metastases. This could indicate the need for standard axillary nodal dissection or other diagnostic and therapeutic approaches, rather than SLN biopsy.

Inflammatory breast cancer is a very aggressive type of breast malignancy involving tumor extension to the dermal lymphatics. The 5-year survival of this subtype of malignancy is reported as low as 10%. Treatment typically involves neoadjuvant chemotherapy, followed by surgical resection and then subsequently adjuvant breast radiation. Staging of this disease is integral to dictate treatment planning. In a recent retrospective study by Carkaci and colleagues[16] from MDACC (M.D. Anderson Cancer Center), PET/CT was shown to improve staging in patients with inflammatory breast cancer. In this study, 41 newly diagnosed patients were investigated with inflammatory breast cancer. PET/CT demonstrated an unusually high percentage of axillary node involvement (90%). The preliminary results of this retrospective study demonstrate that PET/CT shows an exceedingly high percentage of ipsilateral axillary (90%), and subpectoral (44%) nodal disease.[16] Nearly half the patients in the study (49%) had distant metastases at the time of initial staging, and 17% of distant metastatic lesions seen on PET/CT were clinically occult and not evident on baseline imaging.[16] Eleven of the 20 patients (55%) with distant metastases had disease in two or more organ sites.

In conclusion, FDG-PET should not replace axillary node sampling for routine staging of the axilla because even microscopic nodal involvement may be important for prognosis and treatment planning. In addition, PET cannot accurately quantify the number of involved nodes or the presence of extranodal extension because of limited spatial resolution. Quantifying the amount of tumor within the node cannot be determined by PET/CT. However, in certain instances, such as false negative SLNB, or inflammatory breast cancer, PET/CT can provide accurate staging information.

EVALUATION OF EXTRA-AXILLARY DISEASE WITH PET AND PET/CT

Breast cancer can often spread to other regions besides the ipsilateral axilla, including the internal mammary nodes, the superclavicular nodes, and other areas within the mediastinum. As far as distant metastasis, breast cancer most commonly spreads to the bone, lungs, and liver. The current modalities for assessment of these potential sites of disease include contrast tomography for extra-axillary nodal regions, and chest plain film, bone scan, and liver evaluation for distant metastasis. The role of FDG-PET in detecting extra-axillary regional nodal and distant metastases in newly diagnosed breast cancer has been addressed in various studies. Some studies have demonstrated that FDG-PET is superior to conventional diagnostic techniques in the detection of extra-axillary regional nodal metastases particularly to the internal mammary regions during the follow-up period or in cases of advanced disease (**Fig. 4**). Eubank and colleagues[17,18] recently reported that mediastinal and internal mammary lymph node metastases were seen twice as often with FDG-PET as with CT and that the extent of metastases as determined by conventional imaging methods substantially underestimates the stage of the cancer.

In a recent prospective study by Cermik and colleagues,[15] FDG-PET was able to identify regional extra-axillary and distant lesions in the newly diagnosed breast cancer patients with higher sensitivity than with conventional imaging techniques[15]; 9.2% of patients were potentially upstaged because of the findings on FDG-PET scan. This, in turn, would potentially change the surgical treatment plan for many patients.

In a recent prospective study by Fuster and colleagues,[19] 60 patients with biopsy-proven invasive breast cancer whose tumors were greater than 3 cm were staged using PET. The sensitivity and specificity for PET/CT to detect axillary lymph node metastases were 70% and 100%,

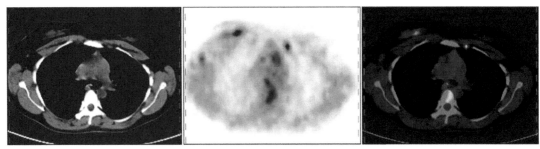

Fig. 4. Axial CT, PET, and PET/CT images of patient who presented with right breast cancer. FDG uptake was noted in right breast primary cancer, right axillary lymph nodes and left internal mammary lymph nodes suggestive of metastatic lymphadenopathy. Postoperative histopathological results confirmed PET/CT findings.

respectively. This figure is similar to the previously quoted numbers regarding tumors of this size. PET was able to detect unsuspected metastatic lesions in the form of extra-axillary nodes (3 of 60 patients), and distant metastases (5 of 60 patients) (**Figs. 5** and **6**). This led to an upstaging of the disease. Additionally, PET/CT detected unexpected infraclavicular node involvement in two patients who were then reclassified as having N3a stage disease.[19] PET/CT also diagnosed one patient with unexpected extra-axillary pathologic nodes located in the supraclavicular region (N3c), and a second patient without proven

disease in the contralateral breast showed a metastatic lymph node in the contralateral axilla.[19] In conclusion, PET/CT led to a change in the initial staging in 42% of patients included in this study, showing higher values of sensitivity and specificity in detecting distant metastases compared with conventional imaging.

In summary, FDG-PET can potentially provide useful staging information in the evaluation of the breast cancer patient. A major advantage is that PET replaces the need for multiple expensive and invasive procedures. Particularly in large primary tumors, PET and PET/CT can potentially

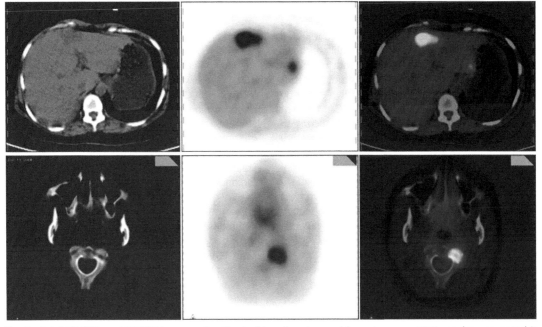

Fig. 5. Axial CT, PET, and PET/CT images of patient of locally advanced breast cancer. FDG uptake was noted in multiple hypodense lesions in multiple segments of liver (*upper row*) and in sclerotic lesion in upper cervical vertebra suggestive of liver and bone metastases.

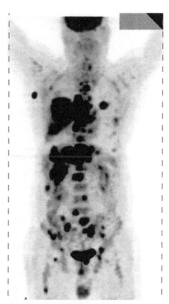

Fig. 6. Whole-body PET projection image of patient of locally advanced breast cancer showing multiple skeletal, lungs, and liver metastases.

upstage the disease and influence treatment planning significantly.

EVALUATING RESPONSE TO NEOADJUVANT TREATMENTS WITH PET AND PET/CT

Neoadjuvant chemotherapy has gained acceptance in treating locally advanced breast cancer. The advantages of neoadjuvant treatment over conventional adjuvant chemotherapy include improved rates of complete resection and the ability to convert mastectomy candidates to breast conservation candidates. The modalities that exist at this time to assess a tumor's response to neoadjuvant treatment include physical exam (PE), MR imaging, and mammography (MG). These three modalities (PE, MG, and MR imaging) have been found to carry both significant false positive and false negative rates.[20–22] In addition, chemotherapy itself may induce significant biologic changes of the tumor, affecting imaging findings differently. As a result, correlation made among MG, MR imaging, PET, and PE findings may not be consistent.

Tumor assessment is important both in planning the initial treatment course and in monitoring disease response to the treatment. Baseline assessment of a palpable breast cancer can dictate the treatment plan either for or against the option of neoadjuvant chemotherapy. If neoadjuvant chemotherapy is selected, monitoring tumor response to treatment by assessing the residual tumor size is essential to determine the best course of surgical action. This evaluation of tumor size is dependent on the relative accuracy of the clinical tools that are used.

In a recent study by Chen and colleagues,[23] CBE (clinical breast examination), MR imaging, and PET were used to assess changes in tumor size during the course of neoadjuvant treatment. Using the PET definition of NR (nonresponder) as less than 50% reduction in tumor SUV, PET was more predictive of pNR (pathologic nonresponder) compared with MR imaging or CBE (**Fig. 7**). Of the six pNR cases, five showed less than 50% SUV reduction (defined as NR) by PET, corresponding to 83% agreement rate between PET and pathology. One of the six cases demonstrated less than 30% tumor size reduction (defined as NR) by CBE, corresponding to 17% agreement rate between CBE and pathology.[23] All of the six pNR cases demonstrated 30% or more tumor size reduction (defined as pathologic or complete response) by MR imaging, corresponding to 0% agreement rate between MR imaging and pathology. Thus, PET helped to reduce the false positive rate of complete and pathologic responders assessed by MR imaging.

Lymph node assessment in patients receiving neoadjuvant chemotherapy can also provide information regarding prognosis as well as treatment planning. In a recent prospective study by Prati and colleagues,[24] the modalities of PE, MG, MR imaging, and PET/CT in tumor and lymph node assessment in patients with T3/T4 tumors receiving neoadjuvant chemotherapy were compared. Forty-five patients received the following chemotherapy regimen: docetaxel/carboplatin with or without trastuzumab before and/or after surgery (depending on human epidermal growth factor receptor 2 [HER-2]/neu status and randomization). Tumor measurements by PE, MG, and MR imaging and lymph node status by PE and PET were obtained before and after neoadjuvant chemotherapy. The results showed PE and PET scan after neoadjuvant chemotherapy to be highly specific for nodal disease, but poor for sensitivity and accuracy. This is comparable to the results reported by Eubank and Mankoff,[25] who also found a sensitivity of 20% and a specificity of 93% for nodal assessment by PET. In addition, baseline PET and PE were shown to be more accurate and sensitive in predicting the final nodal status than the postneoadjuvant evaluation by either PE or PET, but none was sufficient to replace pathologic staging. FDG-PET has the potential to provide valuable staging information and possibly predict tumor response, but its role in the evaluation of lymph node involvement after

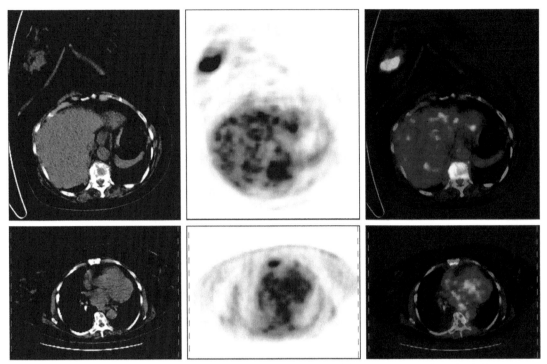

Fig. 7. Axial CT, PET, and PET/CT images of patient of locally advanced breast cancer with multiple bone metastases. Pretherapy (*upper row*) images are showing intense FDG uptake in right breast and vertebral metastasis. Patient was not able to lie down in supine position. Post neoadjuvant chemotherapy (*lower row*) images show resolution of FDG uptake in primary breast cancer and vertebral metastases. Note sclerotic changes in vertebra and sternum, which are usually seen in healed bone metastases.

neoadjuvant chemotherapy has yet to be clearly defined.

In a series of studies conducted by Mankoff and colleagues,[26–29] tumor metabolism as assessed by PET was compared in the setting of neoadjuvant therapy. PET measures of tumor blood flow (BF) and glucose metabolism (FDG K_1) obtained before initiation of neoadjuvant chemotherapy and at midtherapy, predicted response among patients with locally advanced breast cancer. Patients with high pretherapy metabolic blood flow were more likely to have tumors resistant to therapy and were more likely to experience relapse. It was also found that resistant tumors were more likely to have increased blood flow over the course of therapy and that patients whose tumors failed to have a decline in perfusion at midtherapy were more likely to have higher recurrence and mortality risks. These studies also documented that changes in PET measures also predicted the likelihood of achieving a pathologic complete response (pCR) to treatment.

Most recently in 2008, Dunnwald and colleagues[30,31] presented follow-up data to determine whether PET measures of tumor perfusion and metabolism were associated with changes in

survival among patients receiving neoadjuvant chemotherapy. Fifty-three women underwent dynamic [^{18}F] (FDG) and [^{15}O] water PET scans before and at midpoint of neoadjuvant chemotherapy. Patients whose tumors had increases or small reductions in BF and FDG K_1 from pretherapy to midtherapy examinations had elevated recurrence and mortality risks compared with patients with greater reductions in BF and FDG K_1.[30] Additionally, the authors found evidence for higher mortality risk associated with higher BF on midtherapy examinations.

USING PET AND PET/CT TO DETERMINE ESTROGEN RECEPTOR, PROGESTERONE RECEPTOR, AND HER-2 STATUS

Among the various tests for predicting response to treatment, determination of estrogen receptor (ER) and progesterone receptor (PR) in tumor cells is essential for appropriate hormone therapy. The C-erbB-2 (also known as HER-2) receptor has recently been introduced as another predictive and prognostic marker for breast malignancy. Determination of this receptor is useful for selecting patients with advanced breast cancer for treatment with therapeutic antibodies such as trastuzumab (Herceptin; Genentech). In a recent study by Mavi and colleagues,[32] 118 patients with biopsy-proven breast malignancy underwent PET to determine a correlation between SUV and receptor status. ER − lesions had a significantly higher SUVmax than did ER+ lesions (5.64 ± 0.75 versus 3.03 ± 0.26). No interaction was detected between ER and PR states, indicating that the effects of ER and PR states on ^{18}F-FDG uptake are independent of each other.[32] In contrast, two-way analysis of variance (ANOVA) of the ER and C-erbB-2R states showed an interaction between the effects of these receptors. When both these receptors were either positive or negative, the SUVmax was higher than in lesions for which only one receptor was positive. A similar interaction exists between PR state and C-erbB-2R state. These interactions of C-erbB-2R with ER and PR can be interpreted as indicating that the presence or absence of C-erbB-2R reverses the effects of either PR or ER on SUV max measurements. However, neither PR state nor C-erbB-2R state alone had an effect on ^{18}F-FDG uptake. There is also a reverse association between ER and C-erbB-2R indicating that if ER is positive, C-erbB-2R will likely be negative in the malignant tissue. No association was noted between the PR and C-erbB-2R states of these tumors.

PET AND PET/CT IN PREDICTING TUMOR BIOLOGY

Recently, Basu and colleagues[33] compared the SUV values of triple negative tumors (ER −, PR −, HER-2 −) versus ER + PR + HER-2 − tumors. Eighty-eight patients (29 patients with triple-negative breast cancer and 59 patients with ER+/PR+/HER-2− breast cancer) were selected from among 206 individuals with breast carcinoma who were enrolled in the study protocol. For the calculation of FDG-PET characteristics in this group, only those patients who had undergone FDG-PET studies before any intervention were considered. In total, 18 patients in the triple-negative group met these criteria. By following similar criteria, 59 patients with ER+/PR+/HER-2− breast cancer who had focally enhanced uptake of FDG were selected as a control for comparative purposes. For triple-negative cancers, the sensitivity of PET for detecting a lesion was 100%. It was found that stage for stage, tumors from the triple-negative group appeared to have a higher mean SUVmax1 compared with tumors from non–triple-negative control group.[33] Although the

mean SUVmax was higher in the triple-negative group in both tumor size categories, comparison between the two groups demonstrated a statistically significant difference in tumors equal or greater than 2 cm. Basu and colleagues also examined the potential of FDG-PET in predicting tumor biology in a prospective study involving 174 patients with newly diagnosed breast carcinoma at different disease stages who had undergone dual time point FDG-PET before any therapeutic or surgical interventions[34] These patients were divided into three groups: 64 patients with primary and metastatic axillary lymphadenopathy (designated as group I), 18 patients with both axillary and distant metastases (designated as group II), and 92 patients (group III) without any metastasis either at the lymph nodes or at distant sites. The mean SUVmax1, SUVmax2, and the %ΔSUVmax in the early and delayed FDG-PET in group I (n = 64) patients were as follows: primary lesion 4.8% ± 3.9%, 5.3% ± 4.5%, and 9.4% ± 12.8%, respectively, and axillary lesions 3.0% ± 2.6%, 3.0% ± 2.7%, and 1.1% ± 21.3%, respectively. Among the group II patients (n = 18), the mean values of the primary lesion with regard to the SUVmax1, SUVmax2, and the %ΔSUVmax were 7.7% ± 6.2%, 8.9% ± 7.1%, and 15.7% ± 10.8%, respectively. The corresponding figures for the axillary lesions were 3.5% ± 3.1%, 3.7% ± 3.1%, and 6.3% ± 20.9%, respectively, and those for the distant metastatic lesions were 3.0% ± 1.4%, 3.1% ± 1.2%, and 8.5% ± 21.2%, respectively. The mean SUVmax1, SUVmax2, and the %ΔSUVmax of the primary lesion of group III patients (n = 92) without any metastasis were 2.9% ± 2.7%, 3.4% ± 2.4%, and 4.5% ± 4.2%, respectively. Unifactorial ANOVA of the three parameters among the primary lesions of these three groups were statistically significant with regard to the mean SUVmax1 ($P = .01$) and SUVmax2 ($P = .01$). These values in the primary lesions were highest in group II (those with both axillary and distant metastases), followed by group I (those with only metastatic axillary adenopathy) and group III (patients without any metastasis). These results could be related to the more aggressive tumor biology in group II indicating critical information about the behavior of most malignancies at different stages of the disease.[34]

SUMMARY

PET and PET/CT undoubtedly provide useful information regarding prognosis and therapeutic efficacy in the evaluation of breast carcinoma. These modalities are particularly useful in cases of advanced disease, evaluating the response to neoadjuvant chemotherapy, and understanding the biology of different phenotypes of breast cancer. The main limitation of PET and PET/CT in breast cancer is in the detection of small tumors or well-differentiated cancers. With the use of dual point imaging, many of the limitations of specificity can be overcome. Nonetheless, PET and PET/CT remain to be a useful tool in the surgical management of breast malignancy.

REFERENCES

1. Orel SG, Schnall MD. MR imaging of the breast for the detection, diagnosis, and staging of breast cancer. Radiology 2001;220:13–30.
2. Adler LP, Weinberg IN, Bradbury MS. Method for combined FDG-PET and radiographic imaging of primary breast cancers. Breast J 2003;9:163–6.
3. Minn H, Soini I. F-18 fluorodeoxyglucose scintigraphy in diagnosis and follow-up of treatment in advanced breast cancer. Eur J Nucl Med Mol Imaging 1989;15:61–6.
4. Kumar R, Loving VA, Chauhan A, et al. Potential of dual-time-point imaging to improve breast cancer diagnosis with F-FDG PET. J Nucl Med 2005;46:1819–24.
5. Byrne AM, Hill AD, Skehan SJ, et al. Positron emission tomography in the staging and management of breast cancer. Br J Surg 2004.
6. Avril N, Rose CA, Schelling M, et al. Breast imaging with positron emission tomography and fluorine-18 fluorodeoxyglucose: use and limitations. J Clin Oncol 2000;18:3495–502.
7. Wahl RL, Cody RL, Hutchins GD, et al. Primary and metastatic breast carcinoma: initial clinical evaluation with PET with the radiolabled glucose analogue 2-[F-18]-fluoro-2-deoxy-D-glucose. Radiology 1991;179:765–70.
8. Adler LP, Crowe JP, Al-Kaisi NK. Evaluation of breast masses and axillary lymph nodes with [F-18]-2-deoxy-2-fluoro-D-glucose PET. Radiology 1993;187:743–50.
9. Hoh CK, Hawkins RA, Glaspy JA. Cancer detection with whole-body PET using 2-[F-18]-fluoro-2-deoxy-D-glucose. J Comput Assist Tomogr 1993;17:582–9.
10. Mavi A, Urhan M, Yu JQ, et al. Dual time point ^{18}F-FDG PET imaging detects breast cancer with high sensitivity and correlates well with histologic subtypes. J Nucl Med 2006;47:1440–6.
11. Buscombe JR, Holloway B, Roche N, et al. Position of nuclear medicine modalities in the diagnostic work-up of breast cancer. Q J Nucl Med Mol imaging 2004;48(2):109–18.
12. Mabry H, Giuliano AE. Sentinel node mapping for breast cancer: progress to date and prospects for the future. Surg Oncol Clin N Am 2007;16(1):55–70.
13. Lovrics PJ, Chen V, Coates G, et al. A prospective evaluation of positron emission tomography scanning, sentinel lymph node biopsy, and standard axillary dissection for axillary staging in patients with early stage breast cancer. Ann Surg Oncol 2004;11:846–53.
14. Wahl RL, Siegel BA, Coleman RE, et al. Prospective multi-center study of axillary nodal staging with FDG positron emission tomography in breast cancer. J Clin Oncol 2004;22:277–85.
15. Cermik TF, Mavi A, Basu S, et al. Impact of FDG PET on the preoperative staging of newly diagnosed breast cancer. Eur J Nucl Med Mol Imaging 2008;35(3):475–83.
16. Carkaci S, Macapinlac HA, Ristofanilli M, et al. Retrospective study of 18 F–FDG PET/CT in the diagnosis of inflammatory breast cancer: preliminary data. J Nucl Med 2009;50(2):231–8.
17. Eubank WB, Mankoff D, Bhattacharya M, et al. Impact of FDG PET on defining the extent of disease and on the treatment of patients with recurrent or metastatic breast cancer. AJR Am J Roentgenol 2004;183:479–86.
18. De Giorgi U, Valero V, Rohren E, et al. Circulating tumor cells and [18F] fluorodeoxyglucose positron emission tomography/computed tomography for outcome prediction in metastatic breast cancer. J Clin Oncol 2009 May 18.
19. Fuster D, Duch J, Paredes P, et al. Preoperative staging of large primary breast cancer with [18F] fluorodeoxyglucose positron emission tomography/computed tomography compared with conventional imaging procedures. J Clin Oncol 2008;26(29):4746–51.
20. Homer MJ. Mammographic interpretation: a practical approach. New York: McGraw-Hill; 1991. p. 4–5.
21. Orel SG, Schnall MD, LiVolsi VA, et al. Suspicious breast lesions: MR imaging with radiologic-pathologic correlation. Radiology 1994;190:485–93.
22. Mohei M, Abouzied MD, Elpida S, et al. ^{18}F-FDG imaging: pitfalls and artifacts. J Nucl Med Technol 2005;33(3):145–55 2005.
23. Chen Xiaoming, Moore Mark O, Lehman Constance D, et al. Combined use of MRI and PET to monitor response and assess residual disease for locally advanced breast cancer treated with neoadjuvant chemotherapy. Acad Radiol Oct 2004.
24. Prati R, Minami CA, Gornbein JA, et al. Accuracy of clinical evaluation of locally advanced breast cancer in patients receiving neoadjuvant chemotherapy. Cancer 2009;115(6):1194–202.
25. Eubank WB, Mankoff DA. Evolving role of PET in breast cancer imaging. Semin Nucl Med April 2005;35(2):84–99.
26. Mankoff DA, Dunnwald LK, Gralow JR, et al. Changes in blood flow and metabolism in locally

advanced breast cancer treated with neoadjuvant chemotherapy. J Nucl Med 2003;44:1806–14.

27. Ghai S, Muradali D, Bukhanor K, et al. Nonenhancing breast malignancies on MRI: sonographic and pathologic correlation. AJR Am J Roentgenol 2005; 185:481–7.

28. Boetes C, Strijk SP, Holland R, et al. False-negative MR imaging of malignant breast tumors. Eur Radiol 1997;7:1231–4.

29. Teifke A, Hlawatsch A, Beier T, et al. Undetected malignancies of the breast: dynamic contrast-enhanced MR imaging at 1.0T. Radiology 2002; 224:881–8.

30. Dunnwald LK, Gralow JR, Ellis GK, et al. Tumor metabolism and blood flow changes by positron emission tomography: relation to survival in patients treated with neoadjuvant chemotherapy for locally advanced breast cancer. J Clin Oncol 2008;26(27): 4449–57.

31. Mankoff DA, Dunnwald LK, Gralow JR, et al. Blood flow and metabolism in locally advanced breast cancer: relationship to response to therapy. J Nucl Med 2002;43:500–9.

32. Mavi A, Cermik TF, Urhan M, et al. The effects of estrogen, progesterone, and C-erbB-2 receptor states on 18F-FDG uptake of primary breast cancer lesions. J Nucl Med 2007;48(8):1266–72 [Epub 2007 Jul 13. PubMed PMID: 17631558].

33. Basu S, Chen W, Tchou J, et al. Comparison of triple-negative and estrogen receptor-positive/progesterone receptor-positive/HER2-negative breast carcinoma using quantitative fluorine-18 fluorodeoxyglucose/positron emission tomography imaging parameters: a potentially useful method for disease characterization. Cancer 2008;112(5):995–1000.

34. Basu S, Mavi A, Cermik T, et al. Implications of standardized uptake value measurements of the primary lesions in proven cases of breast carcinoma with different degree of disease burden at diagnosis: does 2-deoxy-2-[F-18]fluoro-D-glucose-positron emission tomography predict tumor biology? Mol Imaging Biol 2008;10:62–6.

False-Negative and False-Positive Results in FDG-PET and PET/CT in Breast Cancer

Rakesh Kumar, MD[a],*, Neerja Rani, PhD[b],
Chetan Patel, MD[a], Sandip Basu, MD[c],
Abass Alavi, MD, MD (Hon), PhD (Hon), DSc (Hon)[d]

KEYWORDS

- Breast cancer • Diagnosis • PET/CT • Tumors
- False positive • False negative

Breast cancer is the most frequently diagnosed cancer in women. Approximately 1 in 9 women will have breast cancer during their lifetime. In women worldwide, it remains the second most common cause of cancer death after lung and bronchial cancer. In 2009, it is estimated that 192,370 new cases of breast cancer will be diagnosed among women and 40,170 patients will die from breast cancer in the United States.[1] Although its incidence has increased in the past decades, the overall mortality from this disease has decreased in recent years.[2] In the last decade, along with primary chemotherapy, the treatment of breast cancer has become less radical. Any imaging modality that can be used for the management of breast cancer for initial diagnosis and staging, and to monitor the treatment response, detect recurrences, and predict tumor behavior with high sensitivity and specificity is very useful.

PET/computed tomography (PET/CT) is currently the single most useful diagnostic modality for the management of patients with breast cancer. PET/CT is useful in initial diagnosis, detecting recurrent or metastatic disease, and predicting tumor response to chemotherapy early during treatment. The most important advantage of PET/CT over other imaging techniques is that it provides a high measure of contrast between normal and malignant tissues. Despite many advantages of PET/CT, it has certain shortcomings as an imaging tool for primary breast cancer. A variable sensitivity (range 63%–96%) and specificity (range 75%–100%) of PET and PET/CT in evaluating primary breast lesions has been reported in the literature.[3–8] Most of the initial PET studies done in smaller number of patients and with larger primary breast tumors showed high sensitivity and high specificity of FDG (2-deoxy-2[^{18}F]fluoro-D-glucose)-PET.[3,4] However, recent studies done in breast tumors with smaller size showed relatively lower diagnostic accuracy of PET and PET/CT.[5–8] In this article, the authors discuss various important factors that can lead to false-negative and false-positive results in PET and PET/CT imaging used for the diagnosis of primary breast cancer.

FALSE-NEGATIVE PET AND PET/CT

PET has limited sensitivity in detecting lesions less than 10 mm. PET/CT also cannot detect a lesion beyond the resolution of CT, which is about 4 mm with current PET/CT scanners. Slow-growing and well-differentiated histologic subtypes of breast

---

[a] Department of Nuclear Medicine, All India Institute of Medical Sciences, New Delhi–110029, India
[b] Department of Anatomy, All India Institute of Medical Sciences, New Delhi–110029, India
[c] Radiation Medicine Centre, BARC, Mumbai, India
[d] Nuclear Medicine Section, Radiology Department, Hospital of the University of Pennsylvania, Philadelphia, PA, USA
* Corresponding author.
E-mail address: rkphulia@hotmail.com (R. Kumar).

PET Clin 4 (2009) 289–298
doi:10.1016/j.cpet.2009.09.002

cancer such as tubular carcinoma, lobular carcinoma, and in situ carcinoma show lower FDG uptake than invasive ductal cancer.[5,6] Previous studies have suggested a variety of factors that may affect FDG uptake in breast cancer.[5,6,9–12] **Box 1** shows various factors that can lead to false-negative results on PET and PET/CT imaging.

Tumor Size

Size of the breast lesion is one of the most important factors that determine the sensitivity of FDG-PET and PET/CT in the detection of primary breast cancer. Due to the limited resolution of PET, most of the breast tumors smaller than 10 mm are usually missed by PET. The incorporation of CT with PET led to significant improvement of resolution. The current PET/CT machines have resolutions of approximately 4 mm. However, PET/CT has also limitations in detecting lesions smaller than 4 mm and in situ carcinoma, which is why most of the initial PET studies, which recruited patients with larger primary breast tumors, showed higher diagnostic accuracy compared with PET studies done in patients with smaller primary breast tumors.[3,4] Some investigators found a good correlation between FDG uptake and size of the tumors; however, others could not find any significant correlation between tumor size and FDG uptake.[9,10] Recent studies have shown that standardized uptake value (SUV) decreases as the size of the lesion decreases, which can contribute to higher false-negative rates.[7] Avril and colleagues,[13] in their phantom study, showed a lower detection rate of 28% in lesions smaller than 10 mm. Kumar and colleagues[5] also showed a sensitivity of 23% (7 of 30) in primary breast cancers, which were 10 mm or smaller. In this study, the mean tumor size in false-negative and true-positive lesions was 12.14 ± 13.26 and 20.94 ± 11.80 mm, respectively ($P = 0.003$). There are 3 possible explanations for lower SUVs in small lesions. First, there is a partial volume effect due to the spread of counts over a larger area. Second, an increase in metabolic activity may occur with tumor growth. Third, the breast tumors have lower phosphorylation of FDG than lung cancers.[14]

Box 1
Causes of false-negative PET or PET/CT results

Tumor size

   Less than 10 mm size usually missed by PET
   Less than 4 mm size usually missed by PET/CT

Histologic tumor type

   Lobular carcinomas

   Tubular carcinoma

   Carcinoma in situ

Tumor grade

   Low-grade and well-differentiated tumors

Tumor proliferation

   Low proliferative activity

Tissue heterogeneity

   Lower tumor cell density (necrotic tissue, fibrotic scar, mucinous tumor)

Breast density

   Dense breast may mask small and low-grade tumors

Blood glucose levels

   Uncontrolled blood sugar

   FDG injection without fasting

Data acquisition and data analysis

   Patient movement during the data acquisition

   Supine position (lesion close to chest wall can be missed)

   Respiratory movements lead to blurring of lesion on imaging

---

Histologic Tumor Type

Many investigators have shown that FDG-PET and PET/CT have a higher diagnostic value in patients who have invasive ductal carcinoma (IDC) than in those with invasive lobular carcinoma (ILC) of the breast. In various studies, false-negative results are reported in slow-growing and well-differentiated histologic subtypes of tumors such as tubular carcinoma, in situ carcinoma, and lobular carcinoma. The FDG uptake in ILC was significantly lower than in IDC (mean TBR [Total body radiation] 17.3 vs 6.5, respectively, $P<0.05$),[10] which was attributed to more Ki-67–positive nuclei being present in the ductal subtype compared with lobular breast cancer ($P<0.05$). Similar results were also reported by other investigators.[9,15,16] All these studies found that lobular or tubular subtypes of breast cancer are the common cause of false-negative results. However, in the authors' own study, they were unable to find any correlation between tumor types and false-negative PET results.[5] Although there was no statistically significant correlation between tumor types and false-negative PET results, there were more lobular carcinomas and carcinomas in situ in the false-negative group than in the true-positive group.

Histologic Tumor Grade

Cellular differentiation helps in determining the prognosis of the tumor. High-grade tumors have a poor prognosis and vice versa. FDG uptake is related to pathologic grade of the tumors: lower FDG uptake in differentiated cancers and higher FDG uptake in undifferentiated tumors.[9,10,15] Crippa and colleagues[15] showed that grade 3 breast tumors exhibited higher SUVs of 6.2 than grade 1 and 2 breast tumors, which had a mean SUV of 4.9. This difference in SUVs of different grades of breast tumors was statistically significant. Kumar and colleagues[5] studied 111 patients with breast tumors and reported that patients with true-positive PET results had more high-grade tumors, whereas patients with false-negative PET results had more low-grade tumors (**Fig. 1**) Multivariate logistic regression showed odds of having 16.76 and 6.26 times higher chances of false-negative results with low and moderate grade, respectively, when compared with high-grade tumors ($P = 0.002$ and $P = 0.005$, respectively).

Tumor Proliferation

Tumors with high proliferative activity need more glucose for cell proliferation and energy, and vice versa. This mechanism of higher glucose metabolism in high proliferative tumors can be demonstrated by FDG uptake and Ki-67 expression, and has been shown in studies conducted by Buck and colleagues and Avril and colleagues.[9,10] These investigators showed a significant relation between FDG uptake and Ki-67 expression in ductal breast cancer. However, they did not find any significant relation between FDG uptake and Ki-67 expression in lobular cancer. In contrast to these studies, Crippa and colleagues[15] did not find any relation between SUVs and thymidine labeling index (TLI) of the breast tumors. The contradictory finding of this study can be explained on the basis that Ki-67, which is a monoclonal antibody, helps in determining the proliferative index of breast cancer cells, and its antigen is expressed in G1, S, G2, and M phases of the cell cycle but not in the G0 phase.[17] However, TLI represents only the S-phase fraction.

Tissue Heterogeneity

Most tumor tissue has a heterogeneous cellularity. Malignant cells contribute from a few to more than 90% of the tumor, whereas up to 10% is contributed by inflammatory cells like macrophages, granulation tissue, and necrotic areas. Inflammatory cells and granulation tissue also show increased FDG uptake due to enhanced glucose metabolism in these cells.[18] However, nonmetabolically active components, that is necrotic tissue, fibrotic scar or mucin may reduce FDG uptake in tumors. Therefore, FDG uptake by these cells can affect the overall results of PET imaging. However, Brown and colleagues[19] showed that in mammary cancers in rats, the highest FDG uptake was in areas of highest tumor cell density and lower levels were noted in granulation tissue, necrotic areas, fibrotic regions, and inflammatory cell infiltrates. Kumar and colleagues[7] also found higher FDG uptake in primary breast tumors than postsurgery or excisional biopsy inflammation of breast parenchyma.

Breast Density

A correlation between breast density and FDG uptake has been shown. In a retrospective study, Vranjesevic and colleagues[20] showed that the FDG uptake was significantly higher in dense breast compared with nondense fatty breast. In agreement with these results, the authors' group also found that there was a significant difference in SUVs between the dense and nondense normal breasts.[21,22] Maximum and average SUVs for

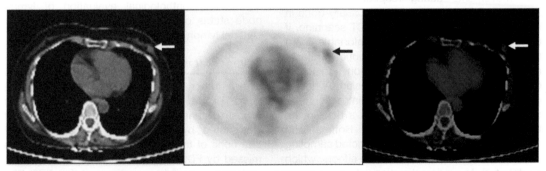

Fig. 1. False-negative PET/CT: Axial section of CT, PET, and PET/CT showing small nodular lesion in outer quadrant of left breast in CT. Mild FDG uptake was noted in PET and PET/CT images (*arrow*). Biopsy of this lesion revealed low-grade ductal carcinoma.

normal tissue of dense breasts were 1.02 ± 0.30 and 0.84 ± 0.27, respectively. Similar values for the nondense breasts were 0.66 ± 0.24 and 0.53 ± 0.23, respectively. There was a significant difference in maximum and average SUVs of breast parenchyma in patients with dense and nondense breasts ($P = .001$). However, the maximum SUVs in the dense breasts were below the threshold of 2.5, a widely used cutoff value for malignancy. However, higher background uptake can considerably affect the visual interpretation of PET and potentially contribute to false-negative reports.

Blood Glucose Levels

FDG uptake in tumor cell cancer is affected by blood glucose levels, as there is competition between the transport of endogenous glucose and FDG molecules. FDG uptake by cancer cells tends to decline as blood glucose and insulin levels increase. Thus, FDG-PET imaging in uncontrolled diabetic patients may lead to false-negative results. In such cases, FDG-PET and PET/CT should be done only if the blood glucose level is less than 200 mg/dL. In patients with uncontrolled diabetes and fasting less than 4 hours, enhanced FDG uptake is noted in cardiac and skeletal muscles.[23] Langen and colleagues[24] found markedly decreased FDG uptake ($41.8\% \pm 15\%$) after glucose infusion in patients with lung cancer. In a similar study, Wahl and colleagues[25] also found that FDG uptake in breast cancer in rats was significantly decreased in hyperglycemia created by continuous glucose infusion. In another study, Wahl and colleagues[3] showed that increasing levels of glucose lead to inhibition of FDG uptake in breast cancer cells.

Data Acquisition and Data Analysis

PET and PET/CT scanning in supine position can cause false-negative results caused by chest wall movements during respiration. Magnetic resonance (MR) breast imaging is usually done in the prone position. PET and PET/CT scanning, if done in prone position on a comfortable foam rubber support, will reduce the motion artifacts and enable better target localization and tracer quantification for primary breast lesion. Avril and colleagues[13] also recommended that patients be scanned in a prone position, with a hole in the foam to ensure breasts hang freely. Hoffman and colleagues[26] observed that the restricted sampling and resolution led to partial volume effects, which contributed to underestimation of local tracer uptake, primarily in tumors smaller than twice the resolution of the imaging system. Thus, correction coefficients are very useful in such scenario, which is mostly obtained from phantom studies.

Axillary Lymph Node Spread

Axillary lymph node metastasis is the single most important factor in determining prognosis and the need for adjuvant chemotherapy.[27] At present, sentinel lymph node biopsy is a well-established procedure for differentiating axillary lymph node metastasis from primary breast cancer.[28,29] This procedure has a high accuracy and can therefore separate those patients who should undergo total axillary dissection, which has high morbidity, from those who can be managed without axillary dissection. Several studies have been performed to investigate the possibility of PET and PET/CT scanning as an independent imaging modality for detecting axillary lymph node status. Most of the recent studies performed in patients with smaller breast tumors showed lower sensitivity of approximately 40%.[30] However, most of these studies showed high specificity in detecting axillary lymph node metastases. Kumar and colleagues[30] found the sensitivity and specificity of FDG-PET for axillary lymph node detection as 44% and 95%, respectively. It was observed that the smallest lymph node detected by PET was 8 mm and that all the micrometastases were missed. These investigators also found that malignancies with moderate and lower histologic grade, lower SUV, and less involvement of lymph nodes resulted in false-negative results. However, no association was found between the size of the primary tumor and false negativity for lymph node spread. Initial studies done with PET in larger primary breast cancer showed relatively high sensitivity and specificity regarding the status of axillary lymph nodes. Many recent studies have yielded conflicting results when the accuracy of FDG-PET was compared with the accuracy of sentinel lymph node biopsy or axillary node dissection.[30–33] It is now clear that FDG-PET and PET/CT cannot replace histopathological evaluation of lymph node status obtained by surgical dissection or sentinel lymph node biopsy.

Distant Metastasis

Breast tumor metastases conforms poor prognosis. Whole body PET scan can be used to assess distant metastases in a single sitting. It was noted by Schirrmeister and colleagues[16] that none of the distant visceral metastases was missed by FDG-PET. However, reports by Cook and colleagues[34] have suggested that FDG-PET is less sensitive in detecting osteoblastic metastases than conventional bone scans. In addition,

FDG-PET has limited application in detecting skull and brain metastases because of high uptake by normal cerebral gray matter.

FALSE-POSITIVE PET AND PET/CT

Whole-body imaging with FDG-PET and PET/CT for the diagnosis, staging, monitoring response to treatment, detection of recurrent malignant diseases is well established. Despite great successes achieved by FDG-PET imaging in the evaluation of malignant disorders, the test is not specific for cancer. Soon after the introduction of FDG-PET for human studies, lesions with substantial inflammatory cells also appeared positive on FDG-PET. Benign processes such as infection, inflammation, and granulomatous diseases seem to increase glycolysis and are therefore readily visualized by FDG-PET imaging. High radiotracer uptake after administration of ^{18}F-FDG corresponds to an increase in glucose uptake and consumption through the hexose monophosphate shunt, which is the main source of energy in chemotaxis and phagocytosis.[35] Activation of phagocytes, also known as respiratory burst activation, leads to increased ^{18}F-FDG uptake.[36] In sterile inflammation, administered ^{18}F-FDG is mainly taken up by neutrophils and macrophages.[37] A high degree of ^{18}F-FDG uptake is seen in neutrophils during the acute phase of inflammation, whereas macrophages and polymorphonuclear leukocytes take up FDG during the chronic phase. **Box 2** shows various factors that can lead to false-positive results on PET and PET/CT imaging.

Benign Breast Lesions

Many benign breast lesions show mild to moderate FDG uptake. Patients with fibrocystic change, atypical ductal hyperplasia, ductal ectasia, and phyllodes tumor may show false-positive findings.[38] On rare occasions gynecomastia can also lead to false-positive results in PET/CT scanning.[39]

Infection and Inflammation

Many infectious and inflammatory breast conditions such as mastitis or abscesses, tuberculosis, fungal infection, and sarcoidosis can lead to false-positive PET or PET/CT results. Alberini and colleagues[40] studied the role of PET/CT imaging in the staging and prognosis of inflammatory breast cancer. PET/CT scan was positive for the primary malignant tumor in 100% and false positive in 2 of 3 patients with benign mastitis. Das and colleagues[41] described a case of disseminated

---

Box 2
Causes of False-positive PET or PET/CT Results

Benign breast lesions
- Ductal hyperplasia/adenoma
- Fibrous dysplasia
- Fibroadenoma
- Gynecomastia
- Fibromatosis
- Florid epitheliosis

Infection and inflammation
- Mastitis/abscesses
- Tuberculosis
- Fungal infection
- Sarcoidosis

Postsurgery
- Post biopsy/lumpectomy/tumorectomy
- Seroma
- Muscle uptake can be seen after surgery because of the distortion of anatomy

Postchemotherapy/Postradiotherapy
- Metabolic flare
- Chemo/ radiotherapy induced inflammation

Mammoplasty/Breast augmentation
- Subsequent changes around prosthesis (foreign substances)
- Ruptured breast implant
- Silicone injection

Posttraumatic
- Hematoma
- Infection/inflammation

Physiologic
- Lactating mothers

---

tuberculosis masquerading as metastatic breast carcinoma on FDG-PET scan in a 37-year old woman. Bakheet and colleagues[42,43] also reported 2 cases of tubercular mastitis showing false-positive uptake of FDG on PET scan. Intense multifocal uptake of FDG in mediastinal, supraclavicular, and para-aortic areas, which were confirmed to represent widespread lymphadenopathy radiologically, was described in mediastinal tuberculosis.[42] Widespread FDG uptake in the mediastinum and retroperitoneum in a patient with known malignancy, which represents widespread lymphadenopathy, can be due to tuberculosis.[42]

Post Surgery

PET and PET/CT have limitations due to false-positive results in evaluation of residual disease activity after biopsy, lumpectomy, or tumorectomy. Increased ^{18}F-FDG-PET is noted as a result of inflammatory changes induced by surgery and radiofrequency ablation.[44] This increased FDG uptake is a result of enhanced inflammatory cell infiltration. Seroma, usually noted after surgery, is a common cause of false-positive results (Fig. 2). Okuma and colleagues[44] showed that neutrophilic infiltration in the alveoli corresponded to a ring-shaped increase in ^{18}F-FDG uptake around the treated area. These changes corresponded to a continuous normalization in ^{18}F-FDG uptake, which takes 6 to 8 weeks. Dual time-point ^{18}F-FDG PET has been suggested to allow for better differentiation between cancer and inflammatory changes. Kumar and colleagues[7] studied 57 breast lesions, of which 39 were malignant and 18 were postbiopsy inflammation. Malignant lesions had an average SUV of 2.87 ± 3.04 whereas in postbiopsy inflammatory lesions SUV averaged 1.28 ± 0.36. If an SUV of 2.5 is considered as cutoff value in differentiating benign and malignant lesions, based on this value only 15 of 39 (38%) lesions will be considered malignant. Kumar and colleagues[7] showed that a percentage change of +3.75 or more in SUV over time (using dual time-point imaging) has high sensitivity and specificity in differentiating inflammatory and malignant lesions. There is an increasing uptake of FDG with time in breast malignancies, whereas the uptake of FDG in inflammatory lesions and normal breast decreases with time.

The PET tracers other than FDG also showed encouraging results. The intracellular accumulation of ^{18}F-fluorothymidine reflects cell proliferation, and ^{18}F-fluorothymidine might be better suited for early detection of persistent or recurrent disease, as no relevant ^{18}F-fluorothymidine uptake was noted in inflammatory lesions.[45] PET tracers targeting angiogenesis might also be suitable to differentiate between residual tumor and treatment-induced inflammation.[46]

In some cases, FDG uptake in muscle can be seen after surgery, because distortion of anatomy can lead to false-positive results on PET or PET/CT. However, this uptake is usually linear and in the course of the muscle. With the introduction of PET/CT, the FDG uptake in muscle can be easily distinguished from pathologic FDG uptake.

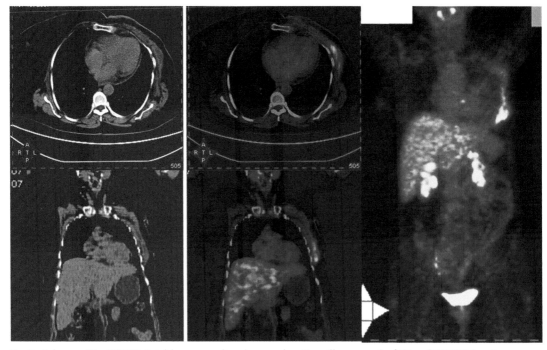

Fig. 2. False-positive PET/CT: Axial (*upper row*) and coronal sections (*lower row*) of CT and PET/CT showing seroma (post surgery) in outer quadrant of left breast in CT. FDG uptake was noted in PET/CT images. Projection PET image (*far left*) also shows intense FDG uptake in left seroma.

Postchemotherapy or Postradiotherapy

PET or PET/CT is frequently being used for the assessment of treatment response, especially in patients with large primary tumors who are receiving neoadjuvant chemotherapy. In responders, a significant decrease in FDG uptake is noted; however, in some cases it has been documented as asynchronous increases in FDG activity, mainly caused by metabolic flare. This phenomenon is commonly seen in bone metastasis. Krupitskaya and colleagues[47] showed this in 4 patients of non-small cell lung cancer who were treated with bevacizumab in addition to standard chemotherapy. All 4 patients developed isolated worsening of their skeletal metastases on PET/CT despite apparent response or stable disease elsewhere.

Postchemotherapy- or postradiotherapy-induced inflammation is not uncommon in patients who receive chemotherapy or radiotherapy. Increased FDG uptake is noted in these patients, caused by enhanced inflammatory cell infiltration (**Fig. 3**). It is recommended that PET or PET/CT scan should be performed only after 4 to 6 weeks of the last cycle of chemotherapy to avoid any false-positive results.

Mammoplasty or Breast Augmentation

Breast augmentation or mammoplasty is not associated with an increased risk for breast cancer; however, breast implants and associated changes around these foreign substances can affect images made by mammography, CT, or MR imaging. PET and PET/CT is said to be free from limitations of conventional imaging. Kobe and colleagues[48] described the features of the PET images of patients who underwent augmentation mammoplasty. Bhargava and colleagues[49] reported inflammatory FDG activity in response to

the ruptured leaking breast prosthesis in a 60-year-old woman. Hurwitz[50] similarly described increased FDG uptake in axillary nodes after ruptured breast prosthesis. Therefore, one should be careful when reporting such cases.

Wahl and colleagues[51] did a feasibility study using FDG-PET imaging in women with silicone-implant augmentation mammoplasties, where mammographic detection of breast cancers is challenging because of the implants' radiodensity, which can obscure tumor visualization. A false increased FDG uptake may be seen in patients with augmentation mammoplasties. Chen and colleagues[52] showed increased FDG uptake in a left breast nodule in a patient with mammoplasty. These investigators showed that FDG-PET could image tumors in the augmented breast without implant displacement and without obvious degradation of image quality by the implant. The patient underwent a left partial mastectomy and the pathology showed a siliconoma.

Posttraumatic

Posttraumatic hematoma and infection or inflammations are also a potential source of false-positive results on FDG-PET or PET/CT scans. As described earlier, increased FDG uptake in such patients is due to increased inflammatory cell infiltration.

Physiologic

High uptake of ^{18}F-FDG in the lactating breast has been reported by many investigators.[53-55] Increased FDG uptake is a result of increased expression of the insulin-independent glucose transporter, GLUT-1, and absence of the insulin-dependent transporter, GLUT-4, in the lactating breast.[55] Four patterns of breast uptake of ^{131}I have been described for the recently lactating breast: full, focal, crescent, and irregular.[56] Similar

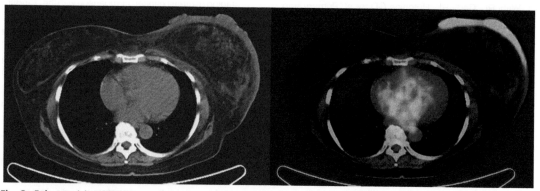

Fig. 3. False-positive PET/CT. Axial sections of CT and PET/CT showing skin thickening and intense FDG uptake in postradiotherapy mastitis.

patterns are also possible on PET or PET/CT scanning in lactating mothers. The glandular uptake of FDG in the breast can mask breast cancer in the postpartum woman undergoing PET scanning.

SUMMARY

Despite the limitations described in this article, ^{18}F-FDG-PET and PET/CT seem to be good modalities in the detection of primary breast cancer. Although MR imaging has better resolution and characterization of small lesions, FDG PET may be useful in prognostication. PET has recently undergone tremendous evolution. PET imaging alone lacks the anatomic landmarks of conventional imaging such as CT and MR imaging; hence, the addition of CT to PET improves detection efficiency and localization of lesions. These images show better specificity and sensitivity than either PET or CT alone. PET mammography is a dedicated tool, which has the added benefits of both anatomic and functional imaging of the breast. PET mammography can detect lesions as small as 5 mm. A combination of PET/MR imaging has the potential added advantage of structural and metabolic delineation of a breast lesion. The role of dual time-point imaging to improve breast cancer diagnosis is also being investigated. Targeted breast imaging using estrogen receptor radioligand is one of the newer scintigraphic techniques, which has an extensive scope in breast cancer detection and treatment monitoring.

REFERENCES

1. Jemal A, Siegel R, Ward E, et al. Cancer statistics, 2009. CA Cancer J Clin 2009;59:225–49.
2. Jemal A, Clegg LX, Elizabeth Ward E, et al. Annual report to the nation on the status of cancer, 1975-2001, with a special feature regarding survival. Cancer 2004;101(1):3–27.
3. Wahl RL, Cody RL, Hutchins GD, et al. Primary and metastatic breast carcinoma: initial clinical evaluation with PET with the radiolabeled glucose analogue 2-[F-18]-fluoro-2-deoxy-D-glucose. Radiology 1991; 179:765–70.
4. Adler LP, Crowe JP, al-Kaisi NK, et al. Evaluation of breast masses and axillary lymph nodes with [F-18] 2-deoxy-2-fluoro-D-glucose PET. Radiology 1993;187:743–50.
5. Kumar R, Chauhan A, Zhuang H, et al. Clinicopathologic factors associated with false negative FDG-PET in primary breast cancer. Breast Cancer Res Treat 2006;98(3):267–74.
6. Avril N, Rose CA, Schelling M, et al. Breast imaging with positron emission tomography and fluorine-18 fluorodeoxyglucose: use and limitations. J Clin Oncol 2000;18:3495–502.
7. Kumar R, Loving V, Chauhan A, et al. Dual time point imaging and its potential to improve breast cancer diagnosis with F18-Fluorodeoxyglucose positron emission tomography. J Nucl Med 2005;46(11): 1819–24.
8. Heusner TA, Kuemmel S, Umutlu L, et al. Breast cancer staging in a single session: whole-body PET/CT mammography. J Nucl Med 2008;49(8): 1215–22.
9. Avril N, Menzel M, Dose J, et al. Glucose metabolism of breast cancer assessed by ^{18}F-FDG PET: histologic and immunohistochemical tissue analysis. J Nucl Med 2001;42:9–16.
10. Buck A, Schirrmeister H, Kuhn T, et al. FDG uptake in breast cancer: correlation with biological and clinical prognostic parameters. Eur J Nucl Med Mol Imaging 2002;29:1317–23.
11. Bos R, van Der Hoeven JJ, van Der Wall E, et al. Biologic correlates of (18)fluorodeoxyglucose uptake in human breast cancer measured by positron emission tomography. J Clin Oncol 2002;20:379–87.
12. Buck AK, Schirrmeister H, Mattfeldt T, et al. Biological characterisation of breast cancer by means of PET. Eur J Nucl Med Mol Imaging 2004; 31(suppl 1):S80–7.
13. Avril N, Bense S, Ziegler SI, et al. Breast imaging with fluorine-18-FDG PET: quantitative image analysis. J Nucl Med 1997;38:1186–91.
14. Torizuka T, Zasadny KR, Recker B, et al. Untreated primary lung and breast cancers: correlation between F-18 FDG kinetic rate constants and findings of in vitro studies. Radiology 1998;207:767–74.
15. Crippa F, Seregni E, Agresti R, et al. Association between [^{18}F] fluorodeoxyglucose uptake and postoperative histopathology, hormone receptor status, thymidine labelling index and p53 in primary breast cancer: a preliminary observation. Eur J Nucl Med 1998;25:1429–34.
16. Schirrmeister H, Kuhn T, Guhlmann A, et al. Fluorine-18 2-deoxy-2-fluoro-D-glucose PET in the preoperative staging of breast cancer: comparison with the standard staging procedures. Eur J Nucl Med 2001;28:351–8.
17. Barnard NJ, Hall PA, Lemoine NR, et al. Proliferative index in breast carcinoma determined in situ by Ki67 immunostaining and its relationship to clinical and pathological variables. J Pathol 1987;152:287–95.
18. Kubota R, Yamada S, Kubota K, et al. Intratumoral distribution of fluorine-18-fluorodeoxyglucose in vivo: high accumulation in macrophages and granulation tissue studied by microautoradiography. J Nucl Med 1992;33:1972–80.
19. Brown RS, Leung JY, Fisher SJ, et al. Intratumoral distribution of tritiated fluorodeoxyglucose in breast carcinoma. I. Are inflammatory cells important? J Nucl Med 1995;36:1854–61.

20. Vranjesevic D, Schiepers C, Silverman DH, et al. Relationship between 18F-FDG uptake and breast density in women with normal breast tissue. J Nucl Med 2003;44:1238–42.

21. Kumar R, Schnall MD, Alavi A. ^{18}F-FDG uptake and breast density in women with normal breast tissue. J Nucl Med 2004;45:1423–4.

22. Kumar R, Chauhan A, Zhuang H, et al. Standardized uptake value in normal breast: effect of age, density and menopausal status. Mol Imaging Biol 2006;8(6): 355–62.

23. Knuuti J, Nuutila P, Ruotsalainen U, et al. Euglycemic hyperinsulinemic clamp and oral glucose load in stimulating myocardial glucose utilization during positron emission tomography. J Nucl Med 1992; 33:1255–62.

24. Langen KJ, Braun U, Kops ER, et al. The influence of plasma glucose levels on fluorine-18-fluorodeoxy-glucose uptake in bronchial carcinomas. J Nucl Med 1993;34:355–9.

25. Wahl RL, Henry CA, Ethier SP. Serum glucose: effects on tumor and normal tissue accumulation of 2-[F-18]-fluoro-2-deoxy-D-glucose FDG in rodents with mammary carcinoma. Radiology 1992;183: 643–7.

26. Hoffmann EJ, Huang S, Phelps ME. Quantitation in positron emission computed tomography: effect of object size. J Comput Assist Tomogr 1979;3: 299–308.

27. Nemoto T, Vana J, Bedwani RN, et al. Management and survival of female breast cancer: results of a national survey by American College of Surgeons. Cancer 1980;45:2917–24.

28. Albertini JJ, Lyman GH, Cox C, et al. Lymphatic mapping and sentinel node biopsy in the patient with breast cancer. JAMA 1996;276:1818–22.

29. Kumar R, Jana S, Heiba SI, et al. Retrospective analysis of sentinel node localization in multicentric palpable and non-palpable breast cance. J Nucl Med 2003;44:7–10.

30. Kumar R, Zhuang H, Schnall M, et al. FDG PET positive lymph nodes are highly predictive of metastasis in breast cancer. Nucl Med Commun 2006;27:231–6.

31. Utech CI, Young CS, Winter PF. Prospective evaluation of fluorine-18 fluorodeoxyglucose positron emission tomography in breast cancer for staging of the axilla related to surgery and immunocytochemistry. Eur J Nucl Med 1996;23:1588–93.

32. van der Hoeven JJ, Hoekstra OS, Comans EF, et al. Determinants of diagnostic performance of [F-18]fluorodeoxyglucose positron emission tomography for axillary staging in breast cancer. Ann Surg 2002;236:619–24.

33. Lovrics PJ, Chen V, Coates G, et al. A prospective evaluation of positron emission tomography scanning, sentinel lymph node biopsy, and standard axillary dissection for axillary staging in patients with early stage breast cancer. Ann Surg Oncol 2004; 11:846–53.

34. Cook GJ, Houston S, Rubens R, et al. Detection of bone metastases in breast cancer by 18-FDG PET: differing metabolic activity in osteoblastic and osteolytic lesions. J Clin Oncol 1998;16:3375–9.

35. Boerman OC, Storm G, Oyen WJ, et al. Sterically stabilized liposomes labeled with indium-111 to image focal infection. J Nucl Med 1995;36:1639–44.

36. Yamada S, Kubota K, Kubota R, et al. High accumulation of fluorine-18-fluorodeoxyglucose in turpentine-induced inflammatory tissue. J Nucl Med 1995;36:1301–6.

37. Kaim AH, Weber B, Kurrer MO, et al. Auto-radiographic quantification of ^{18}F-FDG uptake in experimental soft-tissue abscesses in rats. Radiology 2002;223:446–51.

38. Lim HS, Yoon W, Chung TW, et al. FDG PET/CT for the detection and evaluation of breast diseases: usefulness and limitation. Radiographics 2007; 27(Suppl 1):S197–213.

39. Ramtahalsing R, Arens AI, Vliegen RF, et al. False positive 18F-FDG PET/CT due to gynecomastia. Eur J Nucl Med Mol Imaging 2007;34(4):614.

40. Alberini JL, Lerebours F, Wartski M, et al. ^{18}F-fluoro-deoxyglucose positron emission tomography/computed tomography (FDG-PET/CT) imaging in the staging and prognosis of inflammatory breast cancer. Cancer 2009 [Epub ahead of print].

41. Das CJ, Kumar R, Balakrishnan VB, et al. Disseminated tuberculosis masquerading metastatic breast carcinoma in PET-CT scan. Clin Nucl Med 2008; 33(5):359–61.

42. Bakheet SM, Powe J, Ezzat A, et al. F-18-FDG uptake in tuberculosis. Clin Nucl Med 1998;23(11): 739–42.

43. Bakheet SM, Powe J, Kandil A, et al. F-18 FDG uptake in breast infection and inflammation. Clin Nucl Med 2000;25(2):100–3.

44. Okuma T, Matsuoka T, Okamura T, et al. ^{18}F-FDG small-animal PET for monitoring the therapeutic effect of CT-guided radiofrequency ablation on implanted VX2 lung tumors in rabbits. J Nucl Med 2006;47:1351–8.

45. van Waarde A, Cobben DC, Suurmeijer AJ, et al. Selectivity of ^{18}F-FLT and ^{18}F-FDG for differentiating tumor from inflammation in a rodent model. J Nucl Med 2004;45:695–700.

46. Beer AJ, Haubner R, Goebel M, et al. Biodistribution and pharmacokinetics of the alphav-beta3-selective tracer ^{18}F-galacto-RGD in cancer patients. J Nucl Med 2005;46:1333–41.

47. Krupitskaya Y, Eslamy HK, Nguyen DD, et al. Osteoblastic bone flare on F18-FDG PET in nonsmall cell lung cancer (NSCLC)patients receiving bevacizumab in addition to standard chemotherapy. J Thorac Oncol 2009;4(3):429–31.

48. Kobe K, Chin T, Aoki R, et al. A false-positive fluoro-deoxyglucose positron emission tomography (FDG-PET) imaging result for a patient after augmentation mammoplasty. Aesthetic Plast Surg 2009;33(4): 611–5.

49. Bhargava P, Glass E, Ghesani M. Inflammatory F-18 FDG uptakes secondary to ruptured breast prosthesis. Clin Nucl Med 2006;31(4):227–8.

50. Hurwitz R. F-18 FDG positron emission tomographic imaging in a case of ruptured breast implant: inflammation or recurrent tumor? Clin Nucl Med 2003; 28(9):755–6.

51. Wahl RL, Helvie MA, Chang AE, et al. Detection of breast cancer in women after augmentation mammoplasty using fluorine-18-fluorodeoxyglucose-PET. J Nucl Med 1994;35(5):872–5.

52. Chen CJ, Lee BF, Yao WJ, et al. A false positive F-FDG PET/CT scan caused by breast silicone injection. Korean J Radiol 2009;10(2):194–6.

53. Binns D, Hicks RJ. Pattern of F-18 FDG uptake and excretion in the lactating breast [abstract]. Proceedings of the 9th International PET Conference, San Diego (CA). 1997.

54. Yasuda S, Fujii H, Takahashi W, et al. Lactating breast exhibiting high F-18 FDG uptake. Clin Nucl Med 1998;23:767–8.

55. Hicks RJ, Binns D, Stabin MG. Pattern of uptake and excretion of (18)F-FDG in the lactating breast. J Nucl Med 2001;42(8):1238–42.

56. Bakheet SM, Hammami MM. Patterns of radioiodine uptake by the lactating breast. Eur J Nucl Med 1994; 21:604–8.

Disease Restaging and Diagnosis of Recurrent and Metastatic Disease Following Primary Therapy with FDG-PET Imaging

William B. Eubank, MD[a],*, Jean H. Lee, MD[b],
David A. Mankoff, MD, PhD[b]

KEYWORDS

• FDG PET • PET/CT • Recurrence • Metastases
• Breast cancer • Restaging

Breast cancer is the most common nonskin cancer and the second leading cause of cancer death in women.[1] There are 40,000 women per year dying of breast cancer in the United States, and most breast cancer victims die of progressive metastatic disease.[1] The optimal treatment of patients with recurrent breast cancer depends on knowing the true extent of disease. Conventional imaging (CI) for restaging breast cancer, which includes mammography, ultrasound, and MR imaging for locoregional recurrence (LRR) and contrast-enhanced CT and bone scintigraphy for distant metastasis, covers likely sites of breast cancer recurrence and spread, but may miss sites of recurrence and particularly sites of disease spread. The addition of fluorodeoxyglucose (FDG) PET to CI for detection of recurrent neoplasm after primary treatment of breast cancer has proved to be a complementary imaging technique, overcoming many of the limitations CI for restaging. The additional metabolic information provided by FDG PET increases the accuracy of detecting recurrent or metastatic lesions.[2–16] This is particularly true in the evaluation of extra-axillary regional lymph nodes[2,8,9,11,13,14] and for some bone metastases that are osteolytic.[17–22] Integrated PET-CT systems, with their ability to accurately map foci of elevated FDG uptake to anatomic structures, have provided additional diagnostic confidence and a modest level of accuracy in the evaluation of breast cancer recurrences compared with FDG PET alone.[23–27]

The recognition that breast cancer is a systemic disease, even in its early stages, led to the current approach to treatment, which combines local measures, such as surgery and radiotherapy, with systemic treatment.[28] For most clinical trial studies, local failure is defined as any recurrence of tumor in the ipsilateral chest wall or mastectomy scar; regional failure is defined as any recurrence of tumor in the ipsilateral supraclavicular, infraclavicular, axillary, or internal mammary (IM) nodes;

This work was supported in part by NIH grants RO1CA42045, RO1CA72064, RO1CA90771, and S10RR177229.
a Department of Radiology (S-114-RAD), Puget Sound VA Health Care System, 1660 South Columbian Way, Seattle, WA 98108–1597, USA
b Department of Radiology, University of Washington and Seattle Cancer Care Alliance, Box 356113, Room NN203, 1959 NE Pacific Street, Seattle, WA 98195, USA
* Corresponding author.
E-mail address: weubank@u.washington.edu (W.B. Eubank).

PET Clin 4 (2009) 299–312
doi:10.1016/j.cpet.2009.09.001
1556-8598/09/$ – see front matter. Published by Elsevier Inc.

and recurrence of tumor in any other site is considered as distant failure.[29] In general, systemic therapy is used at almost all disease stages; however, isolated locoregional disease or single sites of metastatic recurrence are also treated with surgery and radiation therapy.[30,31]

The improvement in restaging accuracy for FDG PET and PET-CT compared with CI in patients suspected of having local or distant recurrence has led to changes in treatment strategies in clinical practice.[32,33] This is mostly a result of improved detection of local and distant nodal involvement occult at other imaging studies. The detection of more widespread disease by FDG PET can, particularly in patients thought to have limited locoregional disease based on CI, select patients more appropriately for systemic treatment alone rather than more aggressive, curative treatments, such as surgery and radiation.[33] It is hoped that the potential of FDG PET to provide more accurate and earlier detection of breast cancer recurrences translates into more effective treatment strategies and better health outcomes for these patients in the future.

LOCOREGIONAL RECURRENCES

Recurrence in the breast, skin of the breast, axillary nodes, chest wall, and supraclavicular nodes are the most common sites of first LRR after primary surgical resection.[34] Most LRR occurs within 5 years following primary surgical resection. Although LRR may be an ominous event after mastectomy, data on incidence and outcomes are limited by heterogenous patient populations and the time period studied. Besides extent of primary tumor (size ≥4 cm) and axillary node involvement (four or more positive nodes or extranodal extension), several other risk factors for LRR in postmastectomy patients have been identified.[34] In a large, single-institution retrospective study of patients who underwent mastectomy and multimodality adjuvant treatment,[35] the incidence of LRR was 9% with median 6-year follow-up; multivariate analysis showed age less than 35 years, lymphovascular invasion, and multicentricity as major predictors for isolated LRR. The shift toward breast-conserving surgery and local radiation therapy for early breast cancer in recent years has heightened concern over LRR.[36] The incidence of LRR after breast-conservation treatment ranges from 5% to 22%.[37,38] Independent risk factors associated with LRR in this group of patients include close or positive margins at surgical resection, tumors with extensive intraductal component, high-grade ductal carcinoma in

situ, patient age under 40 years, and absence of radiation after breast-conservation therapy.[37]

LRR involving the chest wall and supraclavicular nodes is associated with poor prognosis in terms of survival after recurrence.[39] For patients presenting with LRR and no evidence of distant disease, however, aggressive multimodality treatment, including surgery, radiation, chemotherapy, and hormonal therapy, may be warranted because many of these patients can be rendered disease-free.[35] Supraclavicular node recurrence is technically considered stage IV disease and generally considered a harbinger to more widely disseminated disease. Patients with supraclavicular node involvement as the sole site of disseminated disease, however, may benefit from aggressive local radiotherapy.[40,41]

The evaluation of local recurrence in the breast, skin, or chest wall with FDG PET can be problematic (**Figs. 1** and **2**). A number of studies evaluating FDG PET and PET-CT have reported both false-positive and false-negative cases of recurrent neoplasm in the skin, residual breast, and chest wall.[7,10,11,24,25,42] Inflammation in these previously treated areas can be a source of FDG avidity, leading to a false-positive result. The tissue volume of some local recurrences may be too small for detection or avidity of the recurrence too low (particularly in cases of lobular carcinoma), leading to a false-negative result.[42] Physical examination and CI, including a combination of mammography, ultrasound, and MR imaging, remains the mainstay for the evaluation of LRR. Because most suspected local recurrences are easily accessible to percutaneous needle biopsy, the definitive status of the suspected lesion can be made by histologic analysis.

A particularly vexing clinical problem occurs in the patient with symptoms of brachial plexopathy suspected of axillary or supraclavicular tumor recurrence, because either tumor recurrence or treatment-induced scarring can be responsible for the symptoms. Hathaway and colleagues[43] showed the value of combining the functional information of FDG PET and the anatomic information from dedicated MR imaging to decide whether patients benefit from further surgery. These results have been confirmed by a subsequent study.[44]

IM AND OTHER EXTRA-AXIAL REGIONAL LYMPH NODE EVALUATION

Lymphatic drainage to the IM nodal chain is an important pathway of spread of disease both at the time of initial diagnosis and after primary treatment of breast cancer. Data from two large sentinel node lymphoscintigraphy series in

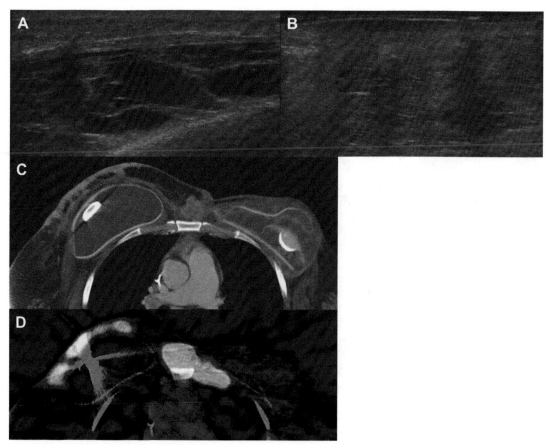

Fig. 1. Recurrence in the contralateral breast in a patient with history of left breast cancer and left partial mastectomy 10 years ago. She also underwent left total mastectomy and prophylactic right mastectomy when she had recurrence 6 years ago. (*A, B*) Ultrasound images show multiple hypoechoic and heterogeneous mixed echogenic lesions with shadowing in the right breast. Axial CT (*C*) and FDG PET-CT images (*D*) reveal hypermetabolic soft tissue mass and nodules with irregular skin thickening in the right breast.

patients with early breast cancer reveal that overall prevalence of drainage to the IM nodes is 17%.[45,46] This is a similar prevalence to that shown in early extended radical mastectomy series where histologically proved metastasis to IM nodes occurred in close to one in five women with operable (stage II–III) breast cancer.[47,48] Metastasis to IM nodes can occur from tumor located anywhere in the breast; however, in the authors' series, IM drainage was significantly less frequent in tumors located in the upper outer quadrant (10%) compared with the other three quadrants and subareolar portion of the breast (17%–29%).[45] Metastasis to the IM and axillary nodes usually occurs synchronously but infrequently (4%–6% incidence) may be isolated to the IM chain.[47]

Neoplastic spread to the IM nodes in axillary node-positive patients is associated with worse prognosis compared with patients only with axillary disease. Early extended radical mastectomy

series showed a significantly worse 10-year overall survival among patients with IM and axillary nodal metastasis (30%) compared with patients having only axillary node disease (55%).[48] Similar prognostic information for drainage to IM nodes at sentinel node lymphoscintigraphy has been shown. Yao and colleagues[46] showed that among axillary node-positive patients with early breast cancer, lymphatic drainage to IM nodes is associated with worse overall survival compared with patients without IM drainage. The IM nodal basins are not routinely sampled because of their relative inaccessibility and their uncertain clinical significance and treatment.[49] Neoplastic involvement of IM nodes may go undetected at initial diagnosis and, if not adequately treated, may give rise to intrathoracic recurrence in the follow-up period. Although the use of FDG PET and PET-CT in detecting IM nodes in early stage disease remains to be proved, a number of studies have pointed toward the value in new or recurrent locally

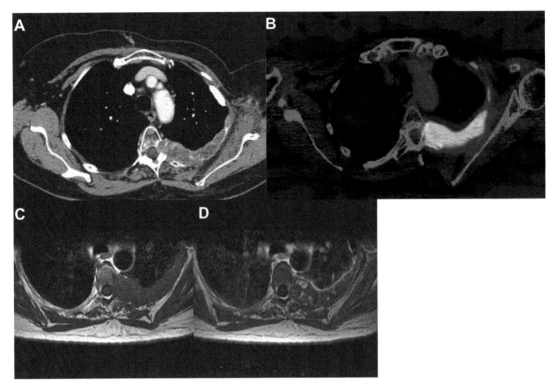

Fig. 2. Locoregional recurrence in the left posterior chest wall in a patient who had undergone left radical mastectomy 13 years ago. She had left anterolateral chest wall recurrence 5 years ago, which had been resected. CT (*A*), FDG PET-CT (*B*), and MR imaging (*C, D*) images show hypermetabolic irregular mass in the left posterior chest wall extending to the epidural space of T5.

advanced breast cancer (LABC).[11,50–52] Experience with imaging patients with LABC shows that the prevalence of IM FDG uptake can be as high as 25% and that the presence of IM FDG uptake predicts treatment failure patterns of disease consistent with IM nodal involvement and progression.[53] A study by Tran and colleagues[54] showed that the likelihood of extra-axillary lymph node findings on FDG PET was affected by the position of the primary tumor (medial versus lateral). The presence of extra-axillary nodal uptake on FDG PET combined with medial tumor location indicated a high risk of subsequent disease progression. These studies suggest that the IM nodal chain is a conduit for more widespread dissemination of disease.

DISTANT METASTASES

FDG PET can be helpful in the evaluation for distant metastases in patients who have been previously treated for their primary disease, particularly in those with advanced stages of disease, equivocal CI findings, and in asymptomatic patients with elevated tumor markers. In terms of diagnostic performance, several studies have

shown FDG PET to have a relative advantage over CI in the evaluation of distant metastases in previously treated patients.[2–11,13,15,16] The largest of these studies are summarized in **Table 1**. In a meta-analysis of FDG PET for the evaluation of breast recurrence and metastases, Isasi and colleagues[55] reported a median sensitivity and specificity of 93% and 82%, respectively, in a patient-based analysis.

A common finding in these studies comparing FDG PET with CI for the detection of recurrent disease is that FDG PET detects a significantly greater number (about twofold) of extra-axial lymph node metastases (**Fig. 3**).[2,8,9,11,13,14] Neoplastic spread to mediastinal nodes is common in patients with advanced disease and as a site of recurrence in patients who have undergone axillary node dissection and radiation. As with IM nodes, mediastinal nodes are rarely sampled in breast cancer patients. CT, the conventional method of staging these nodes, relies on size criteria to determine the presence or absence of disease; this method has been proved significantly less accurate than FDG PET in patients with non–small cell lung cancer where histologic analysis is used as the gold standard.[56,57] In a retrospective series

Table 1
Largest series comparing the ability of whole-body FDG PET with conventional imaging to detect locoregional and distant recurrences in patients who have previously undergone primary treatment for breast cancer

Series	Number of Patients	Confirmed Positive/Negative Cases	% FDG PET Sensitivity (TP/TP + FN)[a]	% FDG PET Specificity (TN/TN + FP)[a]
Bender et al 1997[2]	75	60/15	95 (41/43)	96 (213/221)
Moon et al 1998[3]	57	29/28	93 (27/29)	79 (22/28)
Lonneux et al 2000[4,b]	39	33/6	94 (31/33)	50 (3/6)
Kim et al 2001[5]	27	17/10	94 (16/17)	80 (8/10)
Lin et al 2002[6]	36	11/25	85 (23/27)	96 (85/89)
Liu et al 2002[7,b]	30	28/2	96 (25/28)	50 (1/2)
Suarez et al 2002[8,b]	38	26/12	92 (24/26)	75 (9/12)
Vranjesevic et al 2002[13]	61	42/19	93 (39/42)	84 (16/19)
Gallowitsch et al 2003[9]	62	34/28	97 (33/34)	82 (23/28)
Siggelkow et al 2003[10]	57	31/26	81 (25/31)	98 (25/26)
Kamel et al 2003[11]	60	43/17	89 (24/27) LRR 100 (26/26) DM	84 (16/19) LRR 97 (30/31) DM
Wolfort et al 2006[15]	23	16/7	81 (13/16)	100 (7/7)
Mahner et al 2008[14,c]	119	71/48	87 (62/71)	83 (40/48)

Abbreviations: DM, distant metastases; FN, false negative; FP, false positive; LRR, locoregional recurrence; TN, true negative; TP, true positive.
[a] Values calculated on patient analysis except for Bender and Lin series, which are calculated on lesion analysis.
[b] Patients were mostly or all asymptomatic with elevated tumor markers.
[c] 50/119 patients had undergone primary treatment.

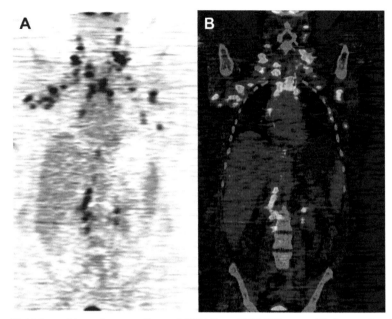

Fig. 3. Patient with history of breast cancer. Coronal PET (*A*) and PET-CT images (*B*) show extensive bilateral axillary, mediastinal, supraclavicular, and retroperitoneal nodal involvement.

of 73 patients with recurrent or metastatic breast cancer who underwent both FDG PET and chest CT,[58] FDG uptake in mediastinal or IM nodes was two times more prevalent than suspiciously enlarged nodes by CT, suggesting that PET is a much more sensitive technique at detecting nodal disease. In the subset of patients with confirmation, the sensitivity of FDG PET was significantly higher (85%) than CT (50%) with nearly the same level of specificity (90% for PET and 83% for CT).

Bone is the most frequent site of recurrence after treatment for primary breast cancer; nearly 70% of patients with advanced disease have skeletal metastases.[59] Metastases from breast cancer can produce a varied physiologic response in bone; lesions can be osteolytic, osteoblastic, or a mixture of the two. Bone scintigraphy has been the standard initial imaging method for the detection of skeletal metastases in oncologic patients because of its ability to survey the entire skeleton with high sensitivity for detection of metastatic lesions. Retrospective studies comparing the sensitivity of bone scintigraphy with FDG PET for the detection of skeletal metastases in patients with advanced breast cancer have shown conflicting results.[3,4,9,14,17–19,60] Some studies have shown FDG PET to be equal or superior to planar bone scintigraphy in the detection of skeletal metastases,[14,18,19] whereas others have shown FDG PET to be less sensitive[3,4,9,60] on a lesion-based analysis. Cook and colleagues[17] were the first investigators to correlate the diagnostic performance of FDG PET and

bone scintigraphy with the morphologic appearance of individual skeletal metastases at plain film radiography or CT. They showed that FDG PET was superior to bone scintigraphy in the detection of osteolytic metastases and bone scintigraphy detected significantly more osteoblastic metastases. Their findings suggest that the physiologic basis of tracer uptake in skeletal metastases with FDG PET and bone scintigraphy is different; FDG uptake is a more direct reflection of metabolically active tumor cells in bone, whereas bone scintigraphy reflects a reparative process occurring in bone tissues adjacent to tumor cells. Cook and colleagues[17] also found that patients with lytic disease had significantly worse survival from time of diagnosis of skeletal metastases than patients with either sclerotic or mixed disease. Others have corroborated these findings,[18–22] leading to the general conclusion that FDG PET and bone scintigraphy are complementary methods for the detection of skeletal metastases in breast cancer patients. These results also suggest that FDG PET and bone scan should not be considered substitutes for each other for skeletal metastasis staging in breast cancer. In the authors' center, bone scintigraphy remains one of the routine studies in breast cancer metastatic staging, with FDG PET to help clarify staging in the case of difficult or equivocal conventional staging.

Evolving data suggest that [F-18]-fluoride PET may improve skeletal metastasis detection compared with bone scintigraphy[61] and may play a role in breast cancer skeletal metastasis staging in the future. Two advantages that [F-18]-fluoride PET has over routine bone scintigraphy are improved image quality because of more favorable pharmacokinetic characteristics and better spatial resolution of PET. [F-18]-fluoride PET has been shown to be more accurate than bone scintigraphy for the detection of both lytic and sclerotic skeletal metastases in oncologic patients.[61,62] In a prospective study comparing [F-18]-fluoride PET with bone scintigraphy in 34 breast cancer patients being evaluated for skeletal metastases, Schirrmeister and colleagues[61] found that [F-18]-fluoride PET was nearly two times more sensitive in detecting metastases and accurately depicted the extent of disease in all 17 patients with proved metastases, whereas 11 out of the 17 patients were undetected with bone scintigraphy. There was also, however, a twofold increase in the detection of benign bone lesions with [F-18]-fluoride PET in this study, raising concern over the potential poor specificity of this modality. Even-Sapir and colleagues[63] showed that this limitation can be overcome with the use of [F-18]-fluoride PET-CT. In their study of 44 oncologic patients, [F-18]-fluoride PET-CT had a significantly better specificity than [F-18]-fluoride PET alone (97% versus 72%). The exact role of [F-18]-fluoride PET and [F-18]-fluoride PET-CT has not yet been determined and is not widely available. It does show promise, however, in making earlier detection of skeletal metastases in breast cancer patients and selecting them for trials of newer therapeutic agents for skeletal metastases that are on the horizon.

The combined PET and CT system has emerged as a routine method of restaging many oncologic patients.[64] In an early retrospective review of 75 breast cancer patients who underwent PET-CT, Tatsumi and colleagues[23] showed PET-CT added incremental diagnostic confidence in 60% of patients who had positive FDG uptake compared with FDG PET alone. The boost in confidence was caused by better anatomic localization of FDG foci in over half of the cases and fewer equivocal readings. The increase in confidence was particularly evident for the evaluation of lymph nodes (57%) and skeletal lesions (77%) in this study. Several of the large retrospective studies of patients being restaged after primary treatment for breast cancer comparing diagnostic performance of PET-CT with either contrast-enhanced CT alone, PET alone, or side-by-side evaluation of CT and PET are summarized in **Table 2**.[23–27,65–67] Fused PET-CT data consistently detected more malignant foci in these studies. On patient-based analysis, however, the studies comparing PET-CT

with PET alone, or side-by-side evaluation of PET and CT, showed marginal (no statistical difference) improvement in sensitivity and specificity for the detection of recurrences. Improvement in accuracy of PET-CT compared with PET alone was caused by[1] better localization of FDG uptake foci, particularly in the mediastinum and cervical regions,[24,25] and in the skeleton[25,26] with a decrease in the number of false-positive findings and an increase in sensitivity to osteoblastic skeletal metastases.[24,26] For the evaluation of pulmonary metastases (**Fig. 4**), there was a tendency for the readers of PET-CT or CT alone to overestimate disease,[24,66,67] probably because any pulmonary nodule seen on CT in this patient group is considered suspicious, and to underestimate disease with PET alone[24,27] because of the small size of these lesions. Slightly fewer hepatic metastases (**Fig. 5**) were detected at CT alone compared with PET-CT or PET alone,[24,26,67] indicating that FDG PET enhances slightly the sensitivity for detecting metastatic disease in the liver. Some investigators have recommended the use of PET-CT for the detection of local and distant recurrences in patients previously treated for primary breast cancer because the combination of CT and PET overcomes the limitations of each modality when used separately.[24,67] This needs to be confirmed in larger prospective trials using FDG-PET-CT–based algorithms.

TREATMENT RESPONSE OF METASTATIC DISEASE

Metastatic breast cancer is often responsive to systemic therapy, and although cure is rarely achieved, with appropriate therapy patients often have prolonged survival and improved quality of life. The use of FDG PET to assess response to treatment has been studied more extensively in the setting of neoadjuvant systemic therapy in patients with LABC[68–70] compared with the metastatic setting.[71–74] As for the assessment of treatment response of LABC, conventional methods used to assess treatment response in metastases, namely whole-body CT or MR imaging and bone scintigraphy, can be problematic. Morphologic changes detected at CT or MR imaging and skeletal scintigraphic abnormalities may persist or be slow to decrease despite good response to systemic therapy. Metabolic imaging with FDG PET has shown promise in making predictions of treatment response or nonresponse earlier and more accurately than CI. Two small prospective studies including patients with multiorgan metastatic disease[71,72] showed that FDG PET was able to accurately predict treatment response as

Table 2
Largest series comparing the ability of PET-CT with FDG PET alone or conventional imaging to detect locoregional and distant recurrences in patients who have previously undergone primary treatment for breast cancer

Series	Number of Patients	Confirmed Positive/ Negative Cases	% PET/CT Sensitivity (TP/TP + FN)[a]	% PET/CT Specificity (TN/TN + FP)[a]	Comparison Imaging
Grahek et al 2004[65,b]	75	57/18	84	78	Physical examination, CI
Fueger et al 2005[26]	58	33/25	94	84	PET alone
Tatsumi et al 2006[23]	69	58/11	84	88	NCCT
Radan et al 2006[66]	46	30/16	90	71	CECT[b]
Haug et al 2007[24,c]	34	26/8	96	89	CECT, PET
Veit-Haibach et al 2007[25]	44	19/25	Correct staging: 91 (N = 40)	Overstaged: 9 (N = 4)	CECT, PET, and PET + CECT
Piperkova et al 2007[67]	34 (restaging) lesions, N = 257	15/19	98	94	CECT
Dirisamer et al 2009[27]	52 lesions, N = 150	42/10	93	100	CECT, PET

Abbreviations: CECT, contrast-enhanced CT; CI, conventional imaging; FN, false negative; FP, false positive; NCCT, noncontrast CT; TN, true negative; TP, true positive.
[a] Values calculated on patient analysis except for Piperkova and Dirisamer series, which are calculated on lesion analysis.
[b] PET gamma camera used.
[c] Fusion software used; all patients were asymptomatic with elevated tumor markers.

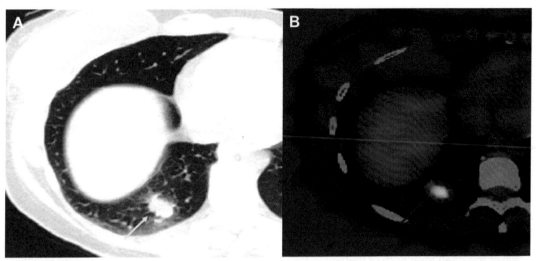

Fig. 4. Pulmonary metastasis in a patient with history of recurrent right breast cancer and widespread metastases to brain and bones. (*A*) CT image shows spiculated nodule in the right lower lobe (*arrow*). (*B*) FDG PET-CT image reveals hypermetabolic activity in the nodule.

early as after the first cycle of chemotherapy, with average decline in lesion standardized uptake value (SUV) of 28% to 42% in responders compared with no change in SUV among nonresponders. Nonresponders were detected earlier than CI during their course of chemotherapy and patients who had no change on follow-up CI were more accurately classified with FDG PET after the first cycle of chemotherapy. In a more recent study of 20 patients with hormone receptor–negative or hormone therapy–refractive

metastatic disease, Couturier and collegues[73] showed that serial FDG PET could accurately predict response to chemotherapy after the third cycle of therapy; SUV decrease was 52% to 56% in responders compared with decrease of 16% to 26% in nonresponders. They found that semiquantitative changes after the first cycle were not predictive, nor was visual assessment at any time point after the start of therapy. FDG PET results following completion of chemotherapy also carry strong prognostic information. In a study

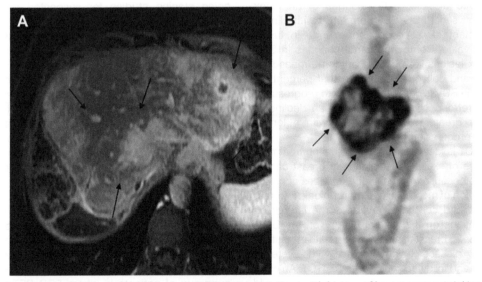

Fig. 5. Recurrence after resection of prior liver metastasis in a patient with history of breast cancer. Axial image of liver MR imaging following gadolinium enhancement (*A*) demonstrates multiple enhancing masses (*arrows*) that correspond to the hypermetabolic activity involving entire liver on coronal FDG PET image (*B*).

of 47 patients with metastatic breast cancer having completed high-dose chemotherapy with autologous stem cell transplantation, Cachin and collegues[75] showed that patients without residual FDG uptake on whole-body scans (complete metabolic response) had significantly longer survival times than those with a positive FDG PET (median survival time 24 months versus 10 months, respectively). The results of these early studies, along with determining the most accurate method of predicting response in the metastatic setting, need to be confirmed in larger prospective trials. The main potential benefit of using FDG PET as a method of assessing treatment response in patients with metastatic breast cancer is the earlier recognition of those who do not respond to systemic chemotherapy, allowing the earlier withdrawal of this often toxic from of therapy.

Because there are many therapeutic options available to patients with skeletal metastases, including local treatment (surgery or radiation) and systemic treatment (chemotherapy, endocrine therapy, diphosphonates, or a combination), accurate assessment of treatment response is crucial to ensure prolonged quality of life and survival. Following patients with bone disease on systemic therapy with serial bone scintigraphy, the standard method, and MR imaging is unsuitable because the disease is not measurable.[76] Tracer uptake on scintigraphy or morphologic change on CT or MR imaging do not accurately represent disease burden[77] or can be misleading as exemplified by the phenomenon of bone scan "flare."[78] In a retrospective study, Stafford and collegues[74] showed that in patients with FDG-positive bone-dominant metastatic disease, SUV changes of an index lesion on serial FDG PET correlated with clinical assessment of response and change in tumor marker value. Comparing serial changes in SUV of index lesions with patient outcome measures, Specht and collegues[79] showed that percentage change in SUV is predictive of time to progression. In this retrospective study, a median decline of 41% or greater was associated with a longer time to progression.

PET-CT is ideally suited for evaluating treatment response of skeletal metastases in breast cancer patients because this technique provides accurate registration of metabolic and morphologic information. Du and collegues[80] made some interesting observations on the natural history of 146 bone lesions in 25 breast cancer patients, with metastatic skeletal disease being treated with systemic therapy and followed serially with PET-CT. An osteoblastic response was seen in most FDG-avid lesions that were either osteolytic (N = 77) or invisible (N = 17) by CT to start with and converted to FDG-negative with additional systemic therapy. The change in CT appearance with additional treatment seems to be helpful, in some cases, in confirming treatment response based on FDG SUV change. Furthermore, Tateishi and collegues[81] showed, in a retrospective study of 102 patients with breast cancer skeletal metastasis undergoing systemic treatment, that a concomitant increase in CT attenuation and decrease in FDG SUV of the index lesion is predictive of a more durable response to therapy. Larger prospective trials are again warranted to confirm these initial observations.

IMPACT ON MANAGEMENT

More important than the diagnostic performance of FDG PET and PET-CT compared with CI is the impact they have on the management of patients with suspected recurrent breast cancer. Unlike patients with some other advanced-stage malignancy, patients with advanced breast cancer can benefit from a variety of therapies including surgery, radiation, chemotherapy, and hormonal therapy. Choosing the most appropriate therapy depends primarily on accurately defining the extent of disease. As of October, 2002, PET has been approved for payment by the Center for Medicare and Medicaid Services in the United States for staging or restaging of patients with recurrent or metastatic disease, especially when conventional staging studies are equivocal. Despite this approval, there is relatively little insight into which patients with recurrent or metastatic breast cancer benefit the most from FDG PET. In a prospective study of 50 women undergoing staging studies for suspected recurrent breast cancer,[32] FDG PET had a significant impact on defining the extent of disease by changing the clinical stage in 36% of patients and on management by inducing changes in therapy in 58% of the patients. In a retrospective study of 125 patients with advanced breast cancer undergoing CI and FDG PET for staging,[33] the extent of disease was changed in 67% (increased in 43% and decreased in 24%) of patients and the therapeutic plan was altered in 32% of patients based on FDG PET findings. Among different referral categories, FDG PET altered therapy most frequently in patients suspected of LRR, under consideration for aggressive local therapy (44%), by demonstrating more widespread disease than expected and avoiding local surgical therapy. Patients with known metastases being evaluated for response to therapy (33%) was another subgroup of patients in whom FDG PET helped the oncologic team make decisions to change therapy. In the authors' study, these two subgroups of patients with advanced disease were most likely to benefit from staging with FDG PET. The more recent retrospective studies comparing PET-CT with contrast-enhanced CT have also shown that PET-CT impacts treatment choices in 20% to 51% of patients.[27,66] The need for a more sensitive staging tool in patients with first-episode LRR was also corroborated by van Oost and collegues[82]; their study of 175 patients showed that 16% had distant metastases at the time of LRR and 24% developed distant metastases within 18 months of confirmation of recurrence. They estimated that FDG PET would upstage and likely change the therapeutic plan in up to 29% of patients with negative conventional staging studies. These results indicate that FDG PET should not be used as the sole restaging tool in patients with recurrent or metastatic disease but to answer specific questions that likely impact their management.

PET-CT also shows promise in radiation treatment planning by modifying target tissue volumes selected for irradiation based on the combination of morphologic and metabolic data.[83] For example, PET-CT may help to further define the supraclavicular or IM nodal region in patients at risk for recurrence in these regions. In a study that included 32 patients with advanced breast cancer and positive FDG uptake in the supraclavicular region,[41] five patients had FDG-positive nodes posterior to the vertebral body transverse process, a location not covered by a typical radiation field to the supraclavicular region and several other patients had nodes close to the medial border of the field. The impact of PET-CT on patient outcomes and which patients benefit from more aggressive radiation coverage needs to be addressed in future studies.

SUMMARY

FDG PET and PET-CT are useful tools for restaging breast cancer patients who have undergone primary therapy, particularly in those with advanced stages, equivocal findings at conventional staging studies, or asymptomatic with elevated tumor markers. In the clinical setting, they should be used to answer specific clinical questions and to complement conventional staging studies, not as a replacement. Evaluation of LRR involving the skin, breast, and chest wall with FDG PET and PET-CT can be problematic because of poor accuracy and diagnosis is usually made by histologic confirmation. For evaluation of distant metastases, FDG PET and PET-CT perform significantly better than conventional staging studies, particularly for the detection of

nodal disease and osteolytic skeletal metastases, and a more accurate method of determining the true extent of disease. One exception is the detection of sclerotic bone metastases; these lesions are not metabolically active enough for FDG PET detection but readily are detected by bone scan. PET-CT enhances diagnostic confidence (with marginal improvement in accuracy) compared with FDG PET alone for the evaluation of metastatic disease. FDG PET and PET-CT can also help in the assessment the treatment response of metastases earlier than CI. Serial FDG PET or PET-CT more accurately reflects disease status in patients with bone-dominant disease undergoing systemic treatment compared with conventional methods.

Preliminary investigations show that FDG PET has the greatest impact on the choice of treatment in patients with suspected or proved LRR who are being considered for aggressive curative treatment and in the evaluation of treatment response in patients with metastatic disease.

REFERENCES

1. Jemal A, Siegel R, Ward E, et al. Cancer statistics, 2008. CA Cancer J Clin 2008;58(2):71–96.
2. Bender H, Kirst J, Palmedo H, et al. Value of [F-18]-fluoro-deoxyglucose positron emission tomography in the staging of recurrent breast carcinoma. Anticancer Res 1997;17(3B):1687–92.
3. Moon DH, Maddahi J, Silverman DH, et al. Accuracy of whole-body [fluorine-18]-FDG PET for the detection of recurrent or metastatic breast carcinoma. J Nucl Med 1998;39(3):431–5.
4. Lonneux M, Borbath II, Berliere M, et al. The place of whole-body PET FDG for the diagnosis of distant recurrence of breast cancer. Clin Positron Imaging 2000;3(2):45–9.
5. Kim TS, Moon WK, Lee DS, et al. Fluorodeoxyglucose positron emission tomography for detection of recurrent or metastatic breast cancer. World J Surg 2001;25(7):829–34.
6. Lin WY, Tsai SC, Cheng KY, et al. [Fluorine-18]-FDG-PET in detecting local recurrence and distant metastases in breast cancer: Taiwanese experiences. Cancer Invest 2002;20(5-6):725–9.
7. Liu CS, Shen YY, Lin CC, et al. Clinical impact of [F-18]-FDG-PET in patients with suspected recurrent breast cancer based on asymptomatically elevated tumor marker serum levels: a preliminary report. Jpn J Clin Oncol 2002;32(7):244–7.
8. Suarez M, Perez-Castejon MJ, Jimenez A, et al. Early diagnosis of recurrent breast cancer with FDG-PET in patients with progressive elevation of serum tumor markers. Q J Nucl Med 2002;46(2): 113–21.

9. Gallowitsch HJ, Kresnik E, Gasser J, et al. [F-18]-fluorodeoxyglucose positron-emission tomography in the diagnosis of tumor recurrence and metastases in the follow-up of patients with breast carcinoma: a comparison to conventional imaging. Invest Radiol 2003;38(5):250–6.

10. Siggelkow W, Zimny M, Faridi A, et al. The value of positron emission tomography in the follow-up for breast cancer. Anticancer Res 2003;23(2C):1859–67.

11. Kamel EM, Wyss MT, Fehr MK, et al. [F-18]-Fluorodeoxyglucose positron emission tomography in patients with suspected recurrence of breast cancer. J Cancer Res Clin Oncol 2003;129(3):147–53.

12. Eubank WB, Mankoff DA, Vesselle HJ, et al. Detection of locoregional and distant recurrences in breast cancer patients by using FDG PET. Radiographics 2002;22(1):5–17.

13. Vranjesevic D, Filmont JE, Meta J, et al. Whole-body [F-18]-FDG PET and conventional imaging for predicting outcome in previously treated breast cancer patients. J Nucl Med 2002;43(3):325–9.

14. Mahner S, Schirrmacher S, Brenner W, et al. Comparison between positron emission tomography using 2-[fluorine-18]-fluoro-2-deoxy-D-glucose, conventional imaging and computed tomography for staging of breast cancer. Ann Oncol 2008;19(7):1249–54.

15. Wolfort RM, Li BD, Johnson LW, et al. The role of whole-body [fluorine-18]-FDG positron emission tomography in the detection of recurrence in symptomatic patients with stages II and III breast cancer. World J Surg 2006;30(8):1422–7.

16. Weir L, Worsley D, Bernstein V. The value of FDG positron emission tomography in the management of patients with breast cancer. Breast J 2005;11(3):204–9.

17. Cook GJ, Houston S, Rubens R, et al. Detection of bone metastases in breast cancer by [F-18]-FDG PET: differing metabolic activity in osteoblastic and osteolytic lesions. J Clin Oncol 1998;16(10):3375–9.

18. Yang SN, Liang JA, Lin FJ, et al. Comparing whole body [F-18]-2-deoxyglucose positron emission tomography and [technetium-99m]-methylene diphosphonate bone scan to detect bone metastases in patients with breast cancer. J Cancer Res Clin Oncol 2002;128(6):325–8.

19. Ohta M, Tokuda Y, Suzuki Y, et al. Whole body PET for the evaluation of bony metastases in patients with breast cancer: comparison with [99mTc]-MDP bone scintigraphy. Nucl Med Commun 2001;22(8):875–9.

20. Abe K, Sasaki M, Kuwabara Y, et al. Comparison of [F-18]-FDG-PET with [99mTc]-HMDP scintigraphy for the detection of bone metastases in patients with breast cancer. Ann Nucl Med 2005;19(7):573–9.

21. Nakai T, Okuyama C, Kubota T, et al. Pitfalls of FDG-PET for the diagnosis of osteoblastic bone metastases in patients with breast cancer. Eur J Nucl Med Mol Imaging 2005;32(11):1253–8.

22. Uematsu T, Yuen S, Yukisawa S, et al. Comparison of FDG PET and SPECT for detection of bone metastases in breast cancer. AJR Am J Roentgenol 2005;184(4):1266–73.

23. Tatsumi MCC, Mortzikos KA, Fishman EK, et al. Initial experience with FDG-PET/CT in the evaluation of breast cancer. Eur J Nucl Med Mol Imaging 2006;33(3):254–62.

24. Haug AR, Schmidt GP, Klingenstein A, et al. [F-18]-fluoro-2-deoxyglucose positron emission tomography/computed tomography in the follow-up of breast cancer with elevated levels of tumor markers. J Comput Assist Tomogr 2007;31(4):629–34.

25. Veit-Haibach P, Antoch G, Beyer T, et al. FDG-PET/CT in restaging of patients with recurrent breast cancer: possible impact on staging and therapy. Br J Radiol 2007;80(955):508–15.

26. Fueger B, Weber WA, Quon A, et al. Performance of 2-deoxy-2-[F-18]-fluoro-D-glucose positron emission tomography and integrated PET/CT in restaged breast cancer patients. Mol Imaging Biol 2005;7:369–76.

27. Dirisamer A, Halpern BS, Flory D, et al. Integrated contrast-enhanced diagnostic whole-body PET/CT as a first-line restaging modality in patients with suspected metastatic recurrence of breast cancer. Eur J Radiol 2009 Jan 30 [Epub ahead of print].

28. Hortobagyi GN. Developments in chemotherapy of breast cancer. Cancer 2000;88(Suppl 12):3073–9.

29. Taghian A, Jeong JH, Mamounas E, et al. Patterns of locoregional failure in patients with operable breast cancer treated by mastectomy and adjuvant chemotherapy with or without tamoxifen and without radiotherapy: results from five National Surgical Adjuvant Breast and Bowel Project randomized clinical trials. J Clin Oncol 2004;22(21):4247–54.

30. Schwaibold F, Fowble BL, Solin LJ, et al. The results of radiation therapy for isolated local regional recurrence after mastectomy. Int J Radiat Oncol Biol Phys 1991;21(2):299–310.

31. Niibe Y, Kuranami M, Matsunaga K, et al. Value of high-dose radiation therapy for isolated osseous metastasis in breast cancer in terms of oligo-recurrence. Anticancer Res 2008;28(6B):3929–31.

32. Yap CS, Seltzer MA, Schiepers C, et al. Impact of whole-body [F-18]-FDG PET on staging and managing patients with breast cancer: the referring physician's perspective. J Nucl Med 2001;42(9):1334–7.

33. Eubank W, Mankoff D, Bhattacharya M, et al. Impact of [F-18]-fluorodeoxyglucose PET on defining the extent of disease and management of patients with

recurrent or metastatic breast cancer. AJR Am J Roentgenol 2004;183:479–86.

34. Katz A, Strom EA, Buchholz TA, et al. Locoregional recurrence patterns after mastectomy and doxorubicin-based chemotherapy: implications for postoperative irradiation. J Clin Oncol 2000;18(15): 2817–27.

35. Buchanan CL, Dorn PL, Fey J, et al. Locoregional recurrence after mastectomy: incidence and outcomes. J Am Coll Surg 2006;203(4):469–74.

36. Fodor J, Major T, Polgar C, et al. Prognosis of patients with local recurrence after mastectomy or conservative surgery for early-stage invasive breast cancer. Breast 2008;17(3):302–8.

37. Huston TL, Simmons RM. Locally recurrent breast cancer after conservation therapy. Am J Surg 2005;189(2):229–35.

38. Touboul E, Buffat L, Belkacemi Y, et al. Local recurrences and distant metastases after breast-conserving surgery and radiation therapy for early breast cancer. Int J Radiat Oncol Biol Phys 1999; 43(1):25–38.

39. Aristei C, Marsella AR, Chionne F, et al. Regional node failure in patients with four or more positive lymph nodes submitted to conservative surgery followed by radiotherapy to the breast. Am J Clin Oncol 2000;23(3):217–21.

40. Chen SC, Chang HK, Lin YC, et al. Prognosis of breast cancer after supraclavicular lymph node metastasis: not a distant metastasis. Ann Surg Oncol 2006;13(11):1457–65.

41. Reed VK, Cavalcanti JL, Strom EA, et al. Risk of subclinical micrometastatic disease in the supraclavicular nodal bed according to the anatomic distribution in patients with advanced breast cancer. Int J Radiat Oncol Biol Phys 2008;71(2):435–40.

42. Heusner TA, Freudenberg LS, Kuehl H, et al. Whole-body PET/CT-mammography for staging breast cancer: initial results. Br J Radiol 2008;81(969): 743–8.

43. Hathaway PB, Mankoff DA, Maravilla KR, et al. The value of combined FDG-PET and magnetic resonance imaging in the evaluation of suspected recurrent local-regional breast cancer: preliminary experience. Radiology 1999;210:807–14.

44. Ahmad A, Barrington S, Maisey M, et al. Use of positron emission tomography in evaluation of brachial plexopathy in breast cancer patients. Br J Cancer 1999;79(3–4):478–82.

45. Byrd DR, Dunnwald LK, Mankoff DA, et al. Internal mammary lymph node drainage patterns in patients with breast cancer documented by breast lymphoscintigraphy. Ann Surg Oncol 2001;8(3):234–40.

46. Yao MS, Kurland BF, Smith AH, et al. Internal mammary nodal chain drainage is a prognostic indicator in axillary node-positive breast cancer. Ann Surg Oncol 2007;14(10):2985–93.

47. Donegan WL. The influence of untreated internal mammary metastases upon the course of mammary cancer. Cancer 1977;39(2):533–8.

48. Veronesi U, Cascinelli N, Greco M, et al. Prognosis of breast cancer patients after mastectomy and dissection of internal mammary nodes. Ann Surg 1985;202(6):702–7.

49. Sugg SL, Ferguson DJ, Posner MC, et al. Should internal mammary nodes be sampled in the sentinel lymph node era? Ann Surg Oncol 2000; 7:188–92.

50. Danforth DN Jr, Aloj L, Carrasquillo JA, et al. The role of [F-18]-FDG-PET in the local/regional evaluation of women with breast cancer. Breast Cancer Res Treat 2002;75(2):135–46.

51. Carkaci S, Macapinlac HA, Cristofanilli M, et al. Retrospective study of [F-18]-FDG PET/CT in the diagnosis of inflammatory breast cancer: preliminary data. J Nucl Med 2009;50(2):231–8.

52. Groheux D, Moretti JL, Baillet G, et al. Effect of [F-18]-FDG PET/CT imaging in patients with clinical stage II and III breast cancer. Int J Radiat Oncol Biol Phys 2008;71(3):695–704.

53. Bellon JR, Livingston RB, Eubank WB, et al. Evaluation of the internal mammary lymph nodes by FDG-PET in locally advanced breast cancer (LABC). Am J Clin Oncol 2004;27(4):407–10.

54. Tran A, Pio BS, Khatibi B, et al. [F-18]-FDG PET for staging breast cancer in patients with inner-quadrant versus outer-quadrant tumors: comparison with long-term clinical outcome. J Nucl Med 2005; 46(9):1455–9.

55. Isasi CR, Moadel RM, Blaufox MD. A meta-analysis of FDG-PET for the evaluation of breast cancer recurrence and metastases. Breast Cancer Res Treat 2005;90(2):105–12.

56. Vansteenkiste JF, Stroobants SG, De Leyn PR, et al. Lymph node staging in non-small-cell lung cancer with FDG-PET scan: a prospective study on 690 lymph node stations from 68 patients. J Clin Oncol 1998;16(6):2142–9.

57. Stroobants S, Verschakelen J, Vansteenkiste J. Value of FDG-PET in the management of non-small cell lung cancer. Eur J Radiol 2003;45(1):49–59.

58. Eubank WB, Mankoff DA, Takasugi J, et al. [F-18]-fluorodeoxyglucose positron emission tomography to detect mediastinal or internal mammary metastases in breast cancer. J Clin Oncol 2001;19(15): 3516–23.

59. Coleman RE, Rubens RD. The clinical course of bone metastases from breast cancer. Br J Cancer 1987;55(1):61–6.

60. Kao CH, Hsieh JF, Tsai SC, et al. Comparison and discrepancy of [F-18]-2-deoxyglucose positron emission tomography and [99m Tc]- MDP bone scan to detect bone metastases. Anticancer Res 2000;20(3B):2189–92.

61. Schirrmeister H, Guhlmann A, Kotzerke J, et al. Early detection and accurate description of extent of metastatic bone disease in breast cancer with fluoride ion and positron emission tomography. J Clin Oncol 1999;17(8):2381–9.

62. Petren-Mallmin M, Andreasson I, Ljunggren O, et al. Skeletal metastases from breast cancer: uptake of [F-18]-fluoride measured with positron emission tomography in correlation with CT. Skeletal Radiol 1998;27(2):72–6.

63. Even-Sapir E, Metser U, Flusser G, et al. Assessment of malignant skeletal disease: initial experience with [F-18]-fluoride PET/CT and comparison between [F-18]-fluoride PET and [F-18]-fluoride PET/CT. J Nucl Med 2004;45(2):272–8.

64. Antoch G, Saoudi N, Kuehl H, et al. Accuracy of whole-body dual-modality [fluorine-18]-2-fluoro-2-deoxy-D-glucose positron emission tomography and computed tomography (FDG-PET/CT) for tumor staging in solid tumors: comparison with CT and PET. J Clin Oncol 2004;22(21):4357–68.

65. Grahek D, Montravers F, Kerrou K, et al. [F-18]-FDG in recurrent breast cancer: diagnostic performances, clinical impact and relevance of induced changes in management. Eur J Nucl Med Mol Imaging 2004;31(2):179–88.

66. Radan L, Ben-Haim S, Bar-Shalom R, et al. The role of FDG-PET/CT in suspected recurrence of breast cancer. Cancer 2006;107:2545–51.

67. Piperkova E, Raphael B, Altinyay ME, et al. Impact of PET/CT in comparison with same day contrast enhanced CT in breast cancer management. Clin Nucl Med 2007;32(6):429–34.

68. Schelling M, Avril N, Nahrig J, et al. Positron emission tomography using [^18F]-fluorodeoxyglucose for monitoring primary chemotherapy in breast cancer. J Clin Oncol 2000;18:1689–95.

69. Mankoff DA, Dunnwald LK, Gralow JR, et al. Blood flow and metabolism in locally advanced breast cancer: relationship to response to therapy. J Nucl Med 2002;43(4):500–9.

70. Schwarz-Dose J, Untch M, Tiling R, et al. Monitoring primary systemic therapy of large and locally advanced breast cancer by using sequential positron emission tomography imaging with [F-18]-fluorodeoxyglucose. J Clin Oncol 2009;27(4):535–41.

71. Gennari A, Donati S, Salvadori B, et al. Role of 2-[F-18]-fluorodeoxyglucose (FDG) positron emission tomography (PET) in the early assessment of response to chemotherapy in metastatic breast cancer patients. Clin Breast Cancer 2000;1(2):62–3 [discussion: 156–6].

72. Dose Schwarz J, Bader M, Jenicke L, et al. Early prediction of response to chemotherapy in metastatic breast cancer using sequential [F-18]-FDG PET. J Nucl Med 2005;46(7):1144–50.

73. Couturier O, Jerusalem G, N'Guyen JM, et al. Sequential positron emission tomography using [F-18]-fluorodeoxyglucose for monitoring response to chemotherapy in metastatic breast cancer. Clin Cancer Res 2006;12(21):6437–43.

74. Stafford SE, Gralow JR, Schubert EK, et al. Use of serial FDG PET to measure the response of bone-dominant breast cancer to therapy. Acad Radiol 2002;9(8):913–21.

75. Cachin F, Prince HM, Hogg A, et al. Powerful prognostic stratification by [F-18]-fluorodeoxyglucose positron emission tomography in patients with metastatic breast cancer treated with high-dose chemotherapy. J Clin Oncol 2006;24(19): 3026–31.

76. Therasse P, Arbuck SG, Eisenhauer EA, et al. New guidelines to evaluate the response to treatment in solid tumors. European Organization for Research and Treatment of Cancer, National Cancer Institute of the United States, National Cancer Institute of Canada. J Natl Cancer Inst 2000;92(3):205–16.

77. Hamaoka T, Madewell JE, Podoloff DA, et al. Bone imaging in metastatic breast cancer. J Clin Oncol 2004;22(14):2942–53.

78. Schneider JA, Divgi CR, Scott AM, et al. Flare on bone scintigraphy following Taxol chemotherapy for metastatic breast cancer. J Nucl Med 1994; 35(11):1748–52.

79. Specht JM, Tam SL, Kurland BF, et al. Serial 2-[F-18]-fluoro-2-deoxy-D-glucose positron emission tomography (FDG-PET) to monitor treatment of bone-dominant metastatic breast cancer predicts time to progression (TTP). Breast Cancer Res Treat 2007;105(1):87–94.

80. Du Y, Cullum I, Illidge TM, et al. Fusion of metabolic function and morphology: sequential [F-18]-fluorodeoxyglucose positron-emission tomography/computed tomography studies yield new insights into the natural history of bone metastases in breast cancer. J Clin Oncol 2007;25(23):3440–7.

81. Tateishi U, Gamez C, Dawood S, et al. Bone metastases in patients with metastatic breast cancer: morphologic and metabolic monitoring of response to systemic therapy with integrated PET/CT. Radiology 2008;247(1):189–96.

82. van Oost FJ, van der Hoeven JJ, Hoekstra OS, et al. Staging in patients with locoregionally recurrent breast cancer: current practice and prospects for positron emission tomography. Eur J Cancer 2004; 40(10):1545–53.

83. Kruser TJ, Bradley KA, Bentzen SM, et al. The impact of hybrid PET-CT scan on overall oncologic management, with a focus on radiotherapy planning: a prospective, blinded study. Technol Cancer Res Treat 2009;8(2):149–58.

Index

Note: Page numbers of article titles are in **boldface** type.

Moving?

Make sure your subscription moves with you!

To notify us of your new address, find your **Clinics Account Number** (located on your mailing label above your name), and contact customer service at:

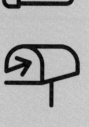

Email: journalscustomerservice-usa@elsevier.com

800-654-2452 (subscribers in the U.S. & Canada)
314-447-8871 (subscribers outside of the U.S. & Canada)

Fax number: 314-447-8029

Elsevier Health Sciences Division
Subscription Customer Service
3251 Riverport Lane
Maryland Heights, MO 63043

Printed and bound by CPI Group (UK) Ltd, Croydon, CR0 4YY

03/10/2024

01040361-0008